Japanese Yumeiho Therapy

a mosaic of oriental therapies

Ranganayakulu Potturu

Professor
Hyderabad, India

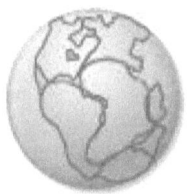

pangea

Amazon, USA
2019

Japanese Yumeiho Therapy
a mosaic of oriental therapies
Author : Dr P.V. Ranganayakulu, India
081427 82241
Published by Amazon, USA
for Pangea Publishers, India
2019

Printed in the United Steates of America

IN MEMORY OF MY TEACHER

MASAYUKI SAIONJI (1943 – 2005)

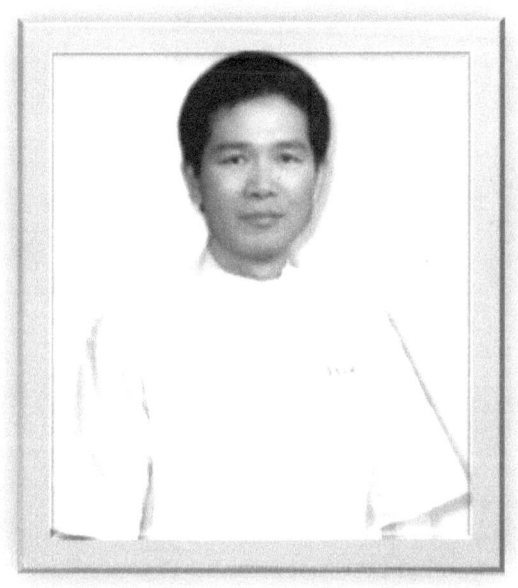

YUMEIHO
骨盤湧命法

Table of Contents

Yoga Fast-forward 6
Masayuki Saionji, the founder 9
Principles of Yumeiho Therapy 12
Tilted Pelvis 21
    Evaluating Hip-Bone Dislocation 26
Hip-correcting Pressing & Kneading Therapy 37
116 Yumeiho Movements 39
    Fundamental Movements 41
    On Spine 49
    On Upper Limbs 58
    On Head & Face 65
    On Lower Limbs 67
    On Abdomen: 79
Indications and Contraindications 84
Frequently Asked Questions 87
Yumeiho across the World 92
YUMEIHO BICS 95
    Standing pose 96
    Sitting posture 109
    Recumbent position 114
Tips for Healthy Skeletal Frame and Muscles 124
Glossary 126

Yoga Fast-forward

I learned Yumeiho therapy in 1994-95 directly from its initiator, Masayuki Saionji at his clinic in Tokyo, Japan. Since then, I applied this therapy on hundreds of patients suffering from various ailments like backache, sciatica and several spine related problems and witnessed good results. I have a long time desire to write a book on theory and practice of Yumeiho therapy. My busy professional life and other assignments have not allowed me to pen my experience with Yumeiho all these years. I teach Ayurveda, the traditional Indian system of medicine and Yumeiho is not part of my profession. Now, after my superannuation from Ayurveda College (University of Health Sciences) in Tirupati, India, find time to review the manuscript for this edition.

I was born and raised in a remote village in south Indian state of Andhra Pradesh. I have not seen an electric bulb or heard a word of another language except my first language Telugu until I was ten years old. After I became a medical doctor in the India's traditional system of medicine, ayurveda – this too on insistence of my father – did not see bright prospects either for this system of medicine or for me. I followed my instincts. I had love for languages, geography, history, astronomy, philosophy, mathematics and anthropology. Books are my best friends. This led me to enter the world of Esperanto, the planned international link language.

Japanese Yumeiho Therapy

My discovery of Yumeiho therapy happened through Esperanto. After learning Esperanto, I travelled to Europe and Far East. Esperantists helped me to explore the world. My varied career included stints as a volunteer at the Universal Esperanto Association in Rotterdam, Netherlands and ayurveda physician at Maharishi Mahesh Yogi's hospital in New Delhi. Later I chose the career of teacher in Sri Venkateswara Ayurveda College run by the famous Hindu religious institution, Tirumala Tirupati Devasthanams in Tirupati, Andhra Pradesh. I became a professor of Ayurveda, the traditional Indian system of medicine.

Once I heard about Yumeiho in 1993, I contacted Dr Masayuki Saionji in Tokyo about my interest to learn this technique. Those were the days of snail mail. He was kind enough to invite me to Tokyo and teach Yumeiho. I visited his clinic named International Institute of Preventive Medicine near the Ueno railway station in Tokyo in two spells (1994 and 1995) for four months. I worked for 8 hours a day to master the technique. He asked me to visit the United States to introduce Yumeiho therapy on the occasion of 43rd Congress of Esperanto League for North America in New York. There I chose the phrase 'Yoga Fast Forward' to interpret the Japanese Yumeiho therapy.

I returned to India with plans of practicing Yumeiho therapy. I applied Yumeiho therapy in my private clinic on hundreds of patients suffering from various complaints ranging from backache to rheumatoid arthritis. The results were always encouraging. However, practicing Yumeiho for years, I felt, is little sickening. I am a traveler. I cannot stay in one field forever! I move on to write a book for enthusiasts. I catch the wonderful opportunity provided by the Amazon to publish books and reach the readers across the world with ease.

As a physician, I know human anatomy and understand the physiological and therapeutic effects of Yumeiho therapy on the human body. I write this book with my two-decade experience of Yumeiho and conviction that this is an economical and effective therapy, which cures and prevents diseases. Moreover, I had the privilege of learning Yumeiho therapy directly from the horse's mouth. I once again thank my guru Dr Masayuki Saionji for hosting me in Tokyo and teaching me his discovery.

This book introduces Yumeiho therapy to the medical professionals and the students of physiotherapy. A picture can explain more than a paragraph of text. This book contains many diagrams because Yumeiho movements are easy to understand through images. The accompanying text of the pictures explains the poses of both therapist and patient without any ambiguity. I thank the International Institute of Preventive Medicine for allowing me to make use of the diagrams used in earlier editions of Yumeiho Therapy by Saionji. I thank my wife Jayalaxmi, who always stands by me.

Ranganayakulu Potturu

Masayuki Saionji, the founder

Masayuki Saionji, born on 18th November 1943 in Tokyo, Japan was destined to synthesize a unique physical therapy from the traditional systems of medicine in Asia. Though interested in medicine, he pursued courses in Commerce in Meiji University upon the insistence of his father. However, he focused more on Chinese language and calligraphy. He discontinued his studies in commerce and became a teacher in calligraphy. He often visited China to improve his technique. There he came in contact with Chinese traditional medicine. In 1975, he met a veteran manual therapist Shuichi Ohno Hidekazu, who is well known for rehabilitation therapy derived from the Chinese Shaolin martial arts. He influenced the life of Saionji forever.

Back in Japan, Saionji studied Shiatsu (finger pressure), a Japanese healing art. Shiatsu is a bodywork derived from so called *anma* method of massage, which was derived from Chinese manual healing art *tui-na*. After graduating from a Shiatsu school, being an innovative person, Saionji invented a new therapy and named it Hip-correcting Pressing and Kneading Therapy or simply YuMeiHo therapy. The word Yumeiho is now under copyright. He founded a Yumeiho clinic in Tokyo, Japan in 1981 and named it International Institute of Preventive Medicine. Saionji authored and published a book *Hipbone Yumeiho Therapy* in 1987 in Japanese and it was translated into 26 languages subsequently. To spread the art across the world, he learned Esperanto, the planned language for international communication, and trained many Esperantists interested in Yumeiho in his clinic. He travelled extensively across the world to teach and treat.

He was a state guest and honorary visiting physician for the Central Military Aviation Hospital in Moscow and treated some cosmonauts suffering from backache. Due to prolonged stays in space labs orbiting the earth at tremendous speeds, some cosmonauts suffer from backache once they reach home. Surprisingly, they are not responding to conventional treatments. Yumeiho was of great help to them. The Central Military Aviation Hospital in Moscow has conducted thorough research on the effects of Yumeiho and published results in Russian language. Dr Saionji has taught Yumeiho to the Russian experts personally during his several visits. He received an honorary PhD from the Russian Ministry of Health.

He received another honorary PhD from San Marino University in Italy. San Marino University uses Esperanto language in curriculum. Between 1989 and 2004, he travelled in more than 40 countries to spread the new art of healing. He visited India in 1996 and presented his technique in the International Conference of the Spinal Surgeons in Coimbatore, in south India. Now, Yumeiho therapists trained in Tokyo practice and teach this technique in 73 countries. His book Yumeiho Therapy published in English, Esperanto, German, French,

Rumanian, Russian, Polish and other languages sold thousands of copies.

Unto his last breath, Masayuki travelled, met new enthusiasts, taught Yumeiho, published articles and books and helped many Esperantists who visited him in Tokyo. He was a generous person and as a true Esperantist loved the world without borders. He had flair for Chinese language, calligraphy and photography. He loves taking pictures of flowers with his camera. His wife and two daughters, who now live in Tokyo, Japan, survive him.

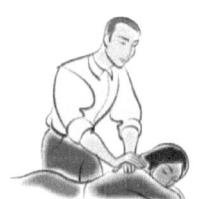

Principles of Yumeiho Therapy

The human body is an amazing machine that evolved to exhibit marvelous faculties and self-awareness. Wheel can be an amazing discovery (axle is an invention) in transportation, however, bipedal or quadruped movement in animals is an impressive way of locomotion. The bipedal movement of the humans allows hands carry objects and keep vision on the horizon. Human bodies appear handsome because they have bilateral symmetry. The bilateral symmetry is caused by the mirror image bones and muscles on both sides. However, several organs are not symmetrical or paired. We have two kidneys, two lungs, two eyes, two ears so on and so forth. However, there is only one stomach, one liver, one pancreas, one heart etc. some solitary organs as brain is symmetrical from left to right. This structure of the body, a slight deviation in anatomical symmetry, renders some physiological imbalance, leading to diseases.

We walk on two legs, which support the pelvic ring. The pelvic girdle, consisting of two hipbones connected each other (anterior) at symphysis pubis and (posterior) to the sacrum at the sacro-iliac joints. This structure forms pelvic ring. The word sacrum really came from sacred because this bone protects the reproductive organs and it is the last one to decompose after death. It endures. The spine, consisting of 33 vertebral bones, provides a canal for descending spinal cord. The sacral and coccyx vertebrae are fused. If the balance on both sides is equal, the hipline, an imaginary straight line that touches the upper ends of right and left hipbones, is horizontal and parallel to the ground.

Similarly, the shoulder line, an imaginary line linking right and left shoulders on the upper side has to be straight and parallel to the hip line. The spine, which is curved anterio-posteriorly, should be straight if viewed from dorsal or ventral directions. However, due to some inherent anatomical asymmetry, habits in locomotion, lopsided weight bearing, gait and posture the hip line, shoulder line and the spine may be deviating from their planes.

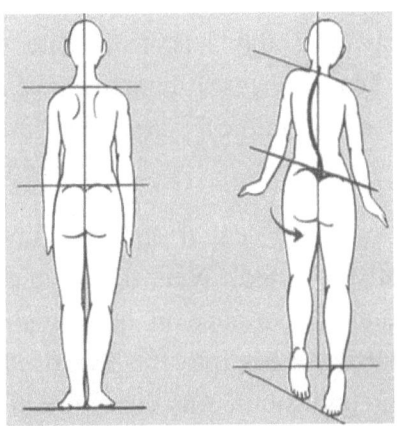

This situation may arise over a long period of time, leading to differences in stretch ability of the muscles. Therefore, some people like to sit legs crossed, left leg over the right leg. They are not comfortable when right leg crosses over left leg. Some tilt the head slightly to right or left. As the spine is not cutting the hipline and shoulder line at right angles, the pelvic girdle is slightly tilted to right or left. This condition ultimately leads to shortening of leg on either side.

The tilting hip girdle is a problem in the bipedals like humans. As the animals walk with four legs, there is no scope for pelvic dislocation. Therefore, four-legged animals hardly suffer from backache and other abnormalities. Animals are healthy as long as they live in the wild. Once they are kept in the zoological gardens and fed regularly, they start suffering from several degenerative diseases. Similarly, humans get their food without much effort at regular intervals; have access to comforts and skip physical exercise, which ultimately lead to a state where humans need more medical services. If humans have active lifestyle and take care of anatomical symmetry, they can lead a healthy life.

What is a big deal if shoulder line, hipline and spine are slightly deviated? Well, the brain and spinal cord are of paramount importance in human physiology. The spinal cord that descends into the spinal cavity gives off spinal nerves on both sides. Any curvature of the spine may slightly press the spinal nerves, which come out in two bundles, anterior ramus and posterior ramus. A neuron, which is physically pressed, adversely affects the muscles and organs it serves.

Japanese Yumeiho Therapy

There is a close relationship between the spine and health status of the human body. The position of the center of gravity of the body can directly influence the health status. The state of the pelvic joints (sacroiliac, coxo-femoral) affects the spine and the body's center of gravity. Thus, anatomical deviations in pelvis may cause functional disorders in the entire organism. Such functional disorders generate, in due course, problems in the locomotive system, serious illnesses of internal organs, nervous system and circulatory system.

The crux of the problem is asymmetry in the skeleton and ensuing rigidity in the muscles. This condition may lead to any pathological conditions depending upon the location of spinal nerve that is compressed or group of muscles that are affected. This asymmetry and loss of equilibrium are corrected manually by Yumeiho therapy.

The body weight, we assume, is born by two legs equally. More than ninety percent of the population has some degree of asymmetry in the musculo-skeletal system. A special weighing machine can measure the difference with two pedals each bearing the weight from one leg. Against popular assumption, the weight of the body is not borne by both legs equally. Yumeiho therapy corrects this asymmetry and establishes equilibrium. To achieve this, Yumeiho employs hundred plus maneuvers.

All these maneuvers are aimed at removing compression on nerves, outstretch muscles, relocate and readjust articulations. Most of the day-to-day health problems are caused by such misalignments in bones and muscles, which can be corrected by appropriate maneuvers. However, why a nerve is compressed and why it causes so much havoc in the body?

Humans have a rigid bony framework inside their bodies, known as endoskeleton. Cockroach has exoskeleton. In humans and animals, bones are joined by articulations (joints) and multiple sacs of lubricants protect the ends of the bones. Muscles, which arise from and insert onto bones ligate the entire body and give us facility of walking and moving. These muscles receive commands from brain. In the human body, nerve cells and muscle cells are the only tissue that is electrically excitable. Nerve cells known as neurons are located in the brain and spinal cord. Several kinds of glial cells, or neuroglia, interlace the neurons for support and nourishment. Thirty-one pairs of spinal nerves exit from the spinal cord from neck to sacrum. Each spinal nerve comes out in two bundles, known as ramii. The anterior ramus contains motor nerve fibers and the posterior ramus contains sensory nerve fibers. Disc herniation or bending of spine engender pinching or entrapment of nerves. Depending on the place of irritation, symptoms manifest.

Neck pain, headache and pain in the face, shoulders, arms and hands may be felt when the nerve is trapped in the neck. Entrapment of nerve may cause numbness or 'pins & needles' in the face, shoulder, arm or hand. Weakness of shoulder, elbow, wrist and diminished hand movements are common.

Pain in the middle of back, chest wall, sternum, and abdomen are due to trapped nerve in the thoracic spine. This may cause numbness or 'pins & needles' in the rib cage or abdomen and may be associated with weakness in the chest and abdomen on one side.

Pain of different intensities in the lower back, buttocks, groin and legs is produced by irritation within the disc itself, or when the disc causes irritation and trapping of the adjacent nerves. If the pain spreads below the knee, we name it Sciatica. It occurs when the nerve becomes increasingly trapped in the lumbar spine. This may cause numbness or pins and needles in the leg and is associated with weakness such as "foot drop" (difficulty in lifting up the toes and foot). Sciatica is a lay term used to describe the pain caused by compression of the spinal nerves. Radiculopathy and radicular pain are the terms used by clinicians.

In the low back, the nerves are most often compressed at L4-L5 and L5-S1. Typically, it is the disc material against the nerve root causes pain to radiate into the buttocks and back of the thigh and calf, and may extend down to the foot. Numbness, tingling, and/or a burning or prickling sensation are common symptoms. If a nerve is compressed in the neck, the symptoms may radiate down the arm.

Peripheral neuropathy, Carpel Tunnel syndrome, Tennis elbow (radial nerve entrapment), Sciatica, Piriformis syndrome are few examples of such pathology. Conventional treatment is aimed at nullifying pain by giving painkillers and steroids to reduce inflammation. Muscle-balance physiotherapy helps patients. Some surgical procedures like microdiscectomy, laminectomy, open decompression, instrumented fusion, and total disc replacement are used to treat these conditions.

However, if a nerve is compressed why it causes so many problems? Such compression diminishes free flow of endoplasm in neuron and obstructs the transmission of impulses leading to weakness in the muscles. Neurons are functional units of brain and spinal cord that are very small but extend over long distances in the body. They propagate impulses using electrochemical energy in the cell. The neuronal connections to the muscles tone them up and make them functional. Sensory neurons carry information from the muscles and other parts of the body that is important to maintain certain tautness in muscles. Motor neurons send impulses to muscles that cause movement. Applying Yumeiho on the muscles also stimulates muscular activity. In such a way Yumeiho therapy aims at establishing symmetry, equal tone of muscles on both sides, releasing entrapped nerves and increasing blood supply into remote places. Yumeiho also stimulates the anti-gravity muscles and muscles least used.

Japanese Yumeiho Therapy

Dr A.P. Kozlovski from Russia opines that the Saionji's method is based on the use of extent of the position change of pelvic bones and spine. Figuratively speaking, the pelvis means foundation and the spine a building on it. In Latin, it is basin or bucket. A smallest vertical deformity occurring in the foundation part of the construction may result in cracks in the wall or in the extreme conditions, the building may ruin. On the analogy of such building, if displacement appears in the pelvic girdle, it will inevitably entail curvature of spine, which in turn has a tangible impact on the vegetative nervous system, circulatory functions and tone of muscles.

The traditional Indian system of medicine, Ayurveda, too has identified the pelvic girdle as the root of bone tissue (*asthidhatu mula*). Yoga, the sibling of Ayurveda proposes several sets of postures aiming equilibrium in the two-legged human body. Practice of Yoga gradually corrects the hipbone dislocation and establishes equilibrium. The practice of Yumeiho therapy may appear as an interdisciplinary between Yoga, physiotherapy, sports medicine and osteopathy.

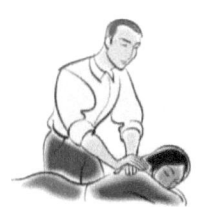

Japanese Yumeiho Therapy

The Human Skeleton

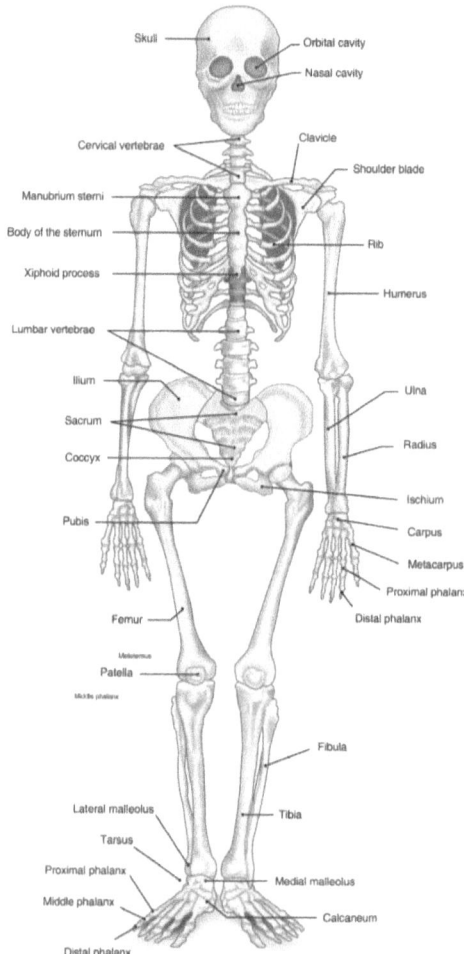

Tilted Pelvis

Before initiating therapy on the patient, the physician has to explore the symmetry of the body and undertake a search for diagnosis. The therapist should examine the patient using the conventional methods like inspection, palpation and interrogation. Take the history of the case and rule out the situations where Yumeiho is of not much help. The therapist should learn to assess the spinal curvature, measure the misalignment of hipline and shoulder line.

Examine the patient closely. The spine or backbone is the key to understand the patient's condition. Let the patient lie with face down i.e. on ventral side. The hands should not be folded but stretched down with palms pointing up and legs medially positioned with toes pointing to median line. A pillow may be used at the chin to support the face. Then, the therapist first examines the row of vertebral/spinal processes on the back. To examine the spine, the patient may remove cloth on the back to see the contour of the spine. Some colored stickers of dots may be fixed on the spinal processes from neck to lower back and see if the spine line is straight. If viewed from left or right, the spine is wavelike i.e. C-shaped at neck, D-shaped at trunk, C-shaped at lumbar region and again D-shaped at sacral level. However, it should be straight in horizontal line if viewed from above. The backbone (spine) is made up of small bones (vertebrae) stacked along with discs in a row. A healthy spine when viewed from left or right sides has gentle curves to it. The curves help the spine absorb stress from body movements. When viewed from the back, in the standing posture, the spine should run straight down from cervical to sacral regions. At the neck, C7, the seventh vertebrae of cervical region, spinal prominence is visible, because this vertebra is anatomically slightly different.

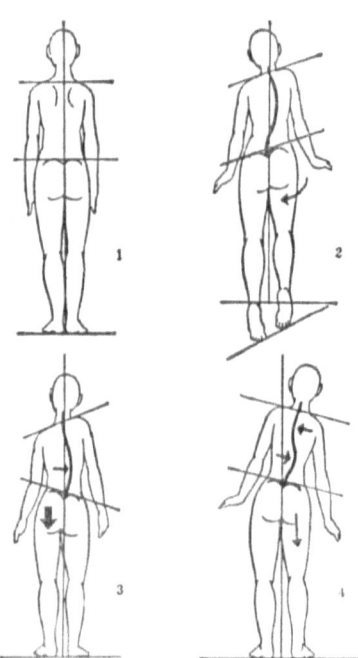

The shoulder line, an imaginary line between two upper parts of shoulders and the hipline, the imaginary line linking two upper locations, Iliac crests in hip girdle, have to be parallel to each other and parallel to the ground. If these two lines are intersected by the vertical spine line, that runs perpendicular to hipline and shoulder line, and cuts at right angles, the spine is in healthy alignment. If the hipline is not horizontal and slightly tilted, it renders either leg slightly longer than the other does.

The therapist sits at feet of the patient, holds two heels with his two hands, and gently pulls along. Then see whether the legs are equal in length. If one leg is slightly longer, it is clearly seen at the unequally positioned at heels when pulled down. In a normal person, the hipline and shoulder line are normal while sitting and standing. However, majority of people have misaligned hipbones. If it is to be corrected, the muscles need good amount of pressing and kneading that keep the bones in proper place. Manipulating joints without press-knead of muscles is not advisable, as the achieved results will not last longer. Here we learn one hundred plus pressing, kneading and joint-readjustment methods, which is known as Hip-Correcting Pressing and Kneading Therapy or simply Yumeiho.

When one side of the body is saddled with more weight than the other, the hipline slightly rises to compensate for imbalance and the hipline inclines from its horizontal position. If the peak of the right hipbone is higher than the left, we reckon it as right hipbone displacement. Similar inclination too can be seen in the shoulder line. These inclinations are observed when a person lies in prone position.

When the right leg is shorter, the left leg weighs more bodyweight. As a result, the thoracic and lumbar vertebrae bend to right and the cervical vertebrae to left to compensate the position change. Anatomical Leg Length Inequality has been extensively researched due to its ripple effect up the lower extremity and spine. 90% of the general population has ALLI variation of 5 mm. If it is more than 20 mm, it may lead to back pain. Proper leg length evaluation is essential before treatment.

The tilted pelvis is a result of sedentary life too. The tilt is not just towards right or left but it could be anterior or posterior. Anterior pelvic tilt and posterior pelvic tilt are easily identified because of gait and pose. There are two sets of muscles that keep the pelvis in its position. The rectus abdominis or simply known as abs, is a paired muscle running vertically on the abdomen. It links pubic symphesis, pubic crest and pubic tubercle to the xiphoid process (lower part of the sternum) and ribs. Three or four bands of connective tissue traverse this muscle pair. In people with low fat, this muscle appears in six-pack or eight pack. The rectus abdominis and abdominal external oblique muscles keep the pelvis in place.

Erector spinea is not just one muscle but a bundle of muscles and tendons that link spine, ribs and pelvis in the back. Iliopsoas is a group of muscles known as dorsal hip muscles or inner hip muscles. Psoas major originates at the thoracic and lumbar vertebrae and associated discs. Iliacus originates in the iliac fossa of the pelvis. Both of these muscles insert into the lesser trochanter of thigh and involved in flexion and lateral rotation of thigh. The greater and lesser trochanters are eminences on the femur bone for muscle attachments.

Rectus abdominus is one of the quadriceps femoris muscle group that link pelvis to the knee. Gluteus is a group of three pairs of muscles that originate in the pelvis and insert into femur. They are responsible for extension, abduction, external rotation and internal rotation of the hip joint.

The hamstring muscles run down the back of the thigh. The three muscles that make up hamstring are Semitendinosus, Semimembranosus and Biceps femoris. They originate at the ischial tuberosity of the pelvis and cross knee joint and end at the lower leg. These muscles help extend leg straight back and bend the knee.

In the anterior pelvic tilt, the pubic bone moves downwards. Whenever this happens, our lumbar curvature is increased. Pelvic tilt to anterior side may happen because of sedentary lifestyle and lack of activity. Anterior rotation of hip gives bad posture to the body. The gluteuls, abdominals and hamstring muscles rotate the hip backwards. The muscles that counter the gluteals, abs and hamstrings should actually neutralize the rotation. However, these muscles may become tight over a period of time. In the posterior tilt, opposite happens. Rise of the pubic bones reduce the lumbar curvature. These movements happen when the pelvis moves around the head of the femur.

Nutation and Counter-nutation terms are used to describe the movement at the sacroiliac joint (SI joint). This is a strong L-shaped synovial joint and bears weight and absorbs shock along with spine. The sacrum articulates with hipbones on both sides. The sacroiliac joints are not fused. An average person will have 3 to 5 millimeters of movement at the sacroiliac joints. This joint too has both internal and external ligaments. As we age, the joint's stability can change and may lose its original orientation. Nutation is the term used to describe movement along an axis. It's the backward rotation of the ilium on the sacrum or anterior and downward movement of the sacrum. Counternutation is opposite to it. This movement has bearing on childbirth. However, too much mobility (hypermobility) or too little mobility (hypomobility) can cause pain. This pain may be radiated to hip, groin, buttocks and back of the thigh. Yumeiho can reduce the inflammation in the sacroiliac joint and reduce pain.

Evaluating Hip-Bone Dislocation

The tilt of the pelvic girdle is visibly recognizable because the skeletal and muscular asymmetry disturbs the anatomical symmetry. Here are the few examples.

Face of the patient is the first place physician starts examining. Closely observed, it gives many signs. One eye may be open more widely than the other may, one eyelid may be partially open, swollen or sunken. Skin folds on the forehead are different from left to right. When eyebrows are raised, folds on forehead may be dissimilar from left to right. One nostril of the nose is little larger than the other. Upon smiling, the face appears asymmetrical i.e. a line may appear on one side of the face.

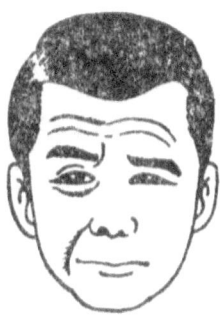

Not just the facial expressions, unconscious movement of the body too reveal about the hipbone dislocation. Any person, who habitually tilts the head to one side, shoulder slightly inclined to one side, hip lifted on either side, the gait is different and unnatural, will have hip dislocation. Toes of one foot may be twisted to one side exhibit skeletal and muscular asymmetry. In some women with hip dislocation, one breast may be slightly smaller than the other. The pose of a person that is naturally assumed clearly indicates the hip tilt.

Indications of Dislocation to Right:

If a person lies in prone position, i.e. chest down, the right hipline is higher than the left. This can be corroborated by palpation. Use your both hands to press and feel the location of iliac crest on both sides and you will feel the right iliac crest is little higher than the left. When you press, the folds formed on the skin on both sides are asymmetrical. As a result, the right leg appears little shorter than the left. When the heels are brought closer, the right heel is higher than the left.

In such right dislocation, blood circulation is affected to the right side and rigidity of musculature follows. When a person with right hip dislocation lies on belly, the left leg instinctively assumes folded position.

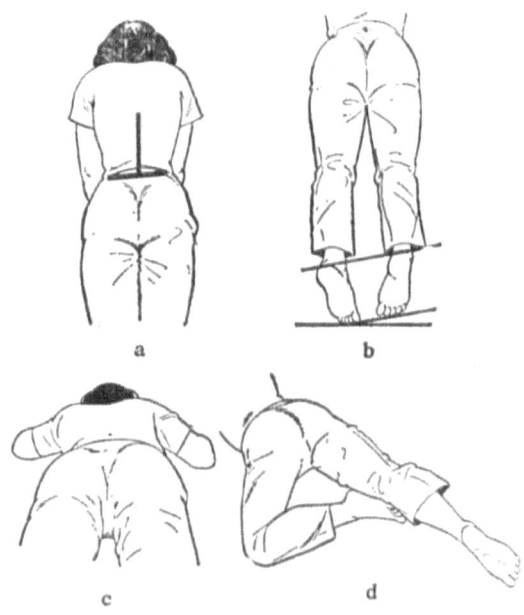

When the patient lies on her back, any of these positions may appear. The left leg is put on the right leg. The right is stretched and the left leg is folded. The left leg turns outside and the left toes are closer to bed while toes of right leg are not closer to bed surface.

When the patient lies on her side, the right leg is under the left leg and crossed.

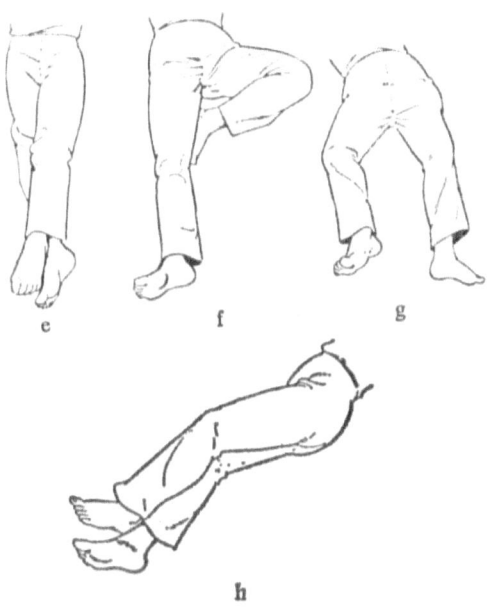

When the patient sits on a chair, the head is slightly tilted to right because the right leg is slightly shorter than the left. This happens to achieve equilibrium in the body. Usually in this condition, the left leg comes before the right leg, when they are crossed. If right leg is put before the left leg in crossing, the patient feels discomfort. If left leg is put on the right leg, the patient does not feel comfortable rather easily gets tired. When both legs are put together, left toes appear little ahead of the right toes. When right and left legs are kept in normal position without crossing, the right leg extends slightly more than the left.

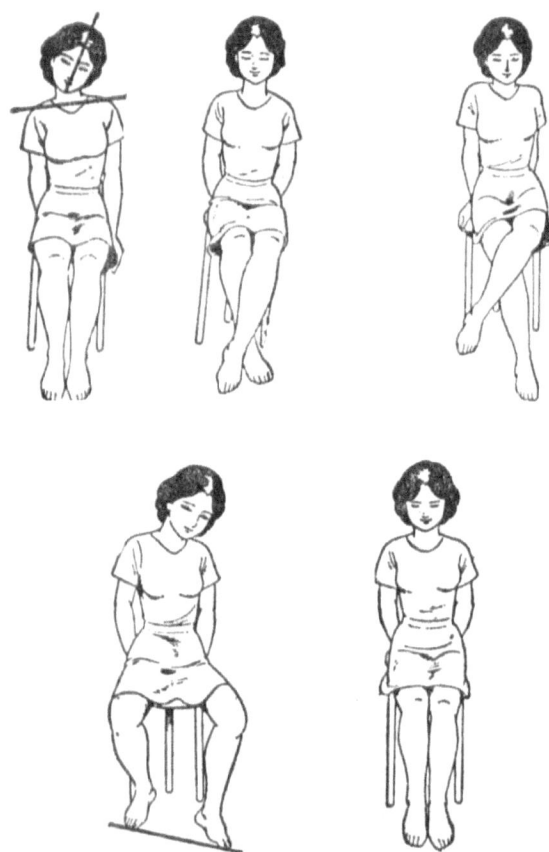

In standing posture, left hip is higher because the right leg is slightly shorter. Therefore, hipline is inclined. While standing they stand on one leg and when tired they shift the weight of the body to the right.

Japanese Yumeiho Therapy

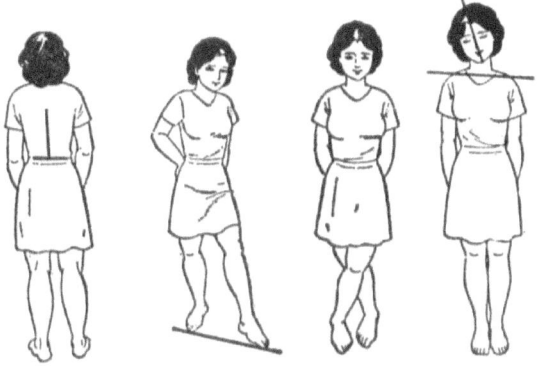

While walking, the spine slightly bends to achieve equilibrium. Subsequently, after a long period, the shoulder too is inclined. In addition, to compensate the balance, head tilts to one side.

Humans are evolved to sit on the floor. Asians are culturally conditioned to sit on the floor. However, on the advent of western culture, use of chairs, upholstered furniture became a common practice across the world. Now the Japanese, Chinese, Indians and other Asians have forgotten to sit on the floor. This leads to several medical conditions.

However, ask the patient to sit on the floor so that you can assess the hip tilt easily. While sitting with both knees bent, the person with hip dislocated to right always keeps the folded legs to left. If folded legs are directed to right, comfort is lacking. If the person sits with folded legs crossed, as shown in the picture, the left leg is shoved into the right leg. Observe the postures of the person while sitting on the floor.

Japanese Yumeiho Therapy

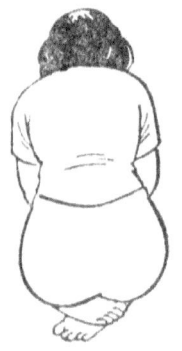

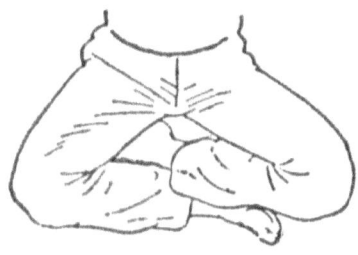

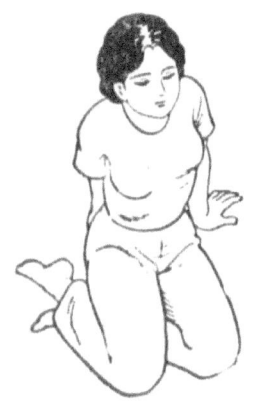

While coming down the stairs, the left leg swings more than the right leg.

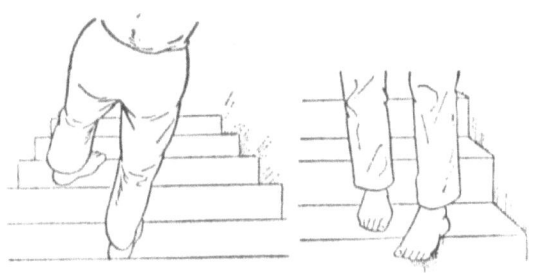

Indications of Dislocation to Left:

In the beginning, the signs of hipbone dislocating to left is identical to the right but we see all the signs explained for right dislocation on the other side. However, both situations may lead to combination kind of thing. Therefore, if clear symptoms of right or left dislocation are not properly seen, the case can be considered as combination type.

Other Signs

Apart from the signs described above, the patients with hipbone dislocation may also show certain variations from right to left, which were observed by Saionji among thousands of patients he treated.

Patients with right dislocation usually do not get obese and are with early gray hair. Patients with left dislocation are usually obese and have more chances of baldhead. The combination type people may become obese after losing weight for some time or may become lean after some period with obesity.

Umbilicus may slightly deviate to right in people with left hip tilt and umbilicus deviates to left in people with right hip tilt. The soles also show differences because one leg is more used than the other is. While squatting or sitting in the toilet, the person extends one leg more than the other does.

In the dislocation of right hipbone, the person extends the fingers of left hand more than its counterpart does. Similarly, the angle between the extended pointing and middle fingers, while making V sign, is more in left hand.

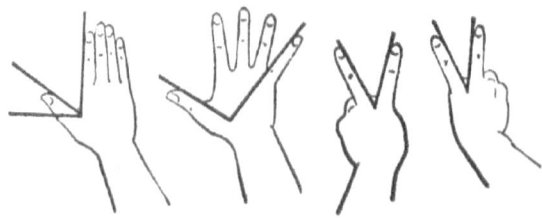

In the dislocation of right hipbone, the big toe of the left foot moves towards the next finger as if it goes below it. All these signs can be seen in reverse order in the dislocation of left hipbone. Observe, these asymmetrical signs are not seen in babies, who have perfectly aligned hip girdle.

Japanese Yumeiho Therapy

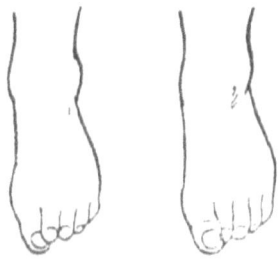

In the persons with dislocation of right hipbone, fingers of right hand and right leg do not crack. If persistently tried, they may crack little. The muscles of the right leg are rigid and stiffer. As the blood circulation is affected in the right side, it affects the fingers and toes on the right side. Therefore, the person shifts the body weight to the left and it worsens the situation. In persons with dislocation of hipbone to the left, similar signs appear on the other side of the body. In combination type, some signs may appear on both sides.

Other signs: Hemicrania (headache on one side), one eye losing its power of clarity in vision, one nostril obstructed frequently, pain on one side of the body etc indicate hip dislocation. When a person bends forward and try to touch the ground, pain is felt either side. See the images in the next page and see how symmetrical your body is. Can you touch your both legs while standing and sitting?

The same posture may be repeated while sitting. If the person can touch one foot and cannot on other side, it indicates the hip dislocation. This is an excellent indication of hip dislocation. The modern medicine too studied in detail about the hiptilt and its effects on vegetative nervous system. Harrison's *Principles of Internal Medicine*, one of the best textbooks on Medicines, gives a detailed chapter on tilted pelvis and outlines pathologies associated with it. However, prescribing appropriate physiotherapy is beyond its purview.

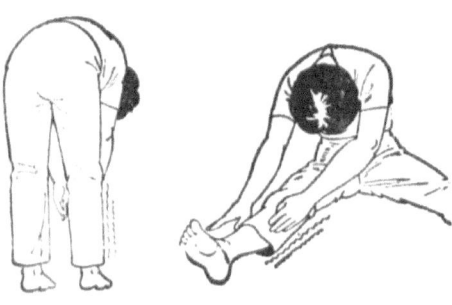

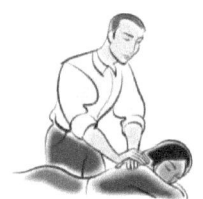

Hip-correcting Pressing & Kneading Therapy

Now, we learn Hip-correcting Pressing and Kneading Therapy or Yumeiho therapy. If this therapy is applied in proper way, it gives immense health benefits. Wrong moves and improper pressure will not solve the problem but may cause undue trauma and damage. Before we start handling the patient, understand the conditions important for both patient and therapist. For successful Yumeiho therapy, proper ambience is important and it boosts the results.

1. The patient wears thin, lightweight and soft clothes. Cotton clothes are better. In this therapy, hands of the therapists do not directly touch the skin of the patient.
2. Upper vest can be removed only if we examine the erectness of the spine on the back. Do not apply this therapy on nude body.
3. Patients remove eyeglasses, wristwatch, shoes, ornaments etc. and arrange for safe custody, while the therapy goes on.
4. The patient has to lie on a thin soft mattress spread on the floor. Doing therapy on a bed or a cot is not possible. A small pillow may be used to support head or chest.
5. The patient has to be relaxed physically and psychologically.
6. While dealing with children, women, senior citizens, obese or lean patients, the therapist has to be careful

enough and understand the flexibility of the joints before using excessive force.

7. The therapist should wear appropriate outfit suitable for free movements.
8. A small pillow may be used under the patient's chest when the patient lies on front.
9. The treatment may be given just one time a day. Each session may continue for 20 minutes.
10. Fifteen to twenty sessions of treatment in a month will reduce rigidity, improve flexibility in the body and symptoms of lethargy subside.
11. The elasticity of each person is different; therefore, the therapist should be cautious and use discretion in delivering pressure on different parts.
12. Deliver force by fingers not by entire hand. This technique is gradually learnt by the therapist.
13. The therapist and the patient need to sit on their knees for short periods during the sessions. Therefore, flexibility is important. Doing Yumeiho also improves the muscle flexibility of the therapist and gives good physical exercise to both.
14. Yumeiho therapy is not advised immediately after lunch or dinner.
15. While dealing with face and head, a thin cloth has to be used to cover the face. Therapist's fingers should not directly touch the face and head of the patient.
16. The therapist and the patient should be barefooted during the session.

116 Yumeiho Movements

Yumeiho therapy consists of 116 manipulations or skillful maneuvers applied on the human body. They help restore anatomical symmetry and physiological equilibrium. By reading this book and looking at the diagrams, it is difficult to remember all these movements. Dr Saionji divides them into two categories. The first category of Fundamental Movements is to be applied on all patients. The second category of maneuvers is to be appropriately applied basing on complaints of the patient. These movements are easy to remember once therapist starts working. We read we forget, we see we remember, we do we understand. It is perfectly applicable to Yumeiho therapy. After you treat some patients, it is easy to remember all 116 manipulations, because by doing memory is enhanced. The best results can be elicited only by mastering all the maneuvers. The skill of the therapist is very important. It accumulates over a period of months and years. In fact, these movements are curative in nature. They help correct dislocated hip-bone alignment and make the spine erect.

These 116 manual twists and turns include some Rolfing or press kneading. They can be broadly divided into two categories. The first category of manipulations is nothing but some press kneading of the muscles and joints. Sixty-four massage-like Rolfing movements are explained along with rest of the 52 realignments of articulations. Rolfing movements are practiced like acupressure technique. Certain muscles are pressed with fingers before we adjust the joints. All the 116 maneuvers are explained here under different headings basing on the area we apply these techniques like upper limbs, lower limbs, abdomen, spine, head and neck. This chapter begins with certain fundamental movements, important to explore the symmetry of the body and to make corrections. These movements are useful for all patients with any kinds of signs and symptoms.

When joints are stretched, cracking or popping sounds appear. We experience this when we do knuckle-cracking. Earlier, physiologists thought knuckles and joints crack when pressed due to popping of bubbles in the synovial fluid that are formed in articulations. New research suggests that this long-held theory may be wrong. Researchers used MRI video to determine why joints make popping sounds when they crack. Rather than being caused by bubbles popping, sound comes from a gas-filled cavity (bubble) forming. As the joint surfaces suddenly separate, there is no more fluid available to fill the increasing joint volume, so a cavity is created and that is associated with sound. Cracking is quite normal and it is a physiological process. This is not associated with arthritis. Our joints are surrounded by synovial membrane, which forms a capsule around the ends of bones. Inside this membrane is synovial fluid, which acts as lubricant and shock absorber so our bones don't grind together when we move. Although cracking is normal, you are not advised to crack the knuckles or joints frequently. Frequent cracking is even harmful for those who are suffering from osteoarthritis.

Cracking sounds may also be caused by tendons, which keep muscles attached to bones, and ligaments. When they slop over joints while moving similar sounds appear, however they do not indicate any pathology. We may often crack out our fingers and feel refreshed. However, cracking sounds always do not mean that the muscles and connective tissue have softened sufficiently.

Before initiating Yumeiho therapy, assure that all the requirements are fulfilled. Good ambience is important. Let the patient and therapist are in relaxed mood.

Fundamental Movements

The patient lies on belly with face and palms facing ground. The therapist sits at the feet of the patient on heels and holds the ankles. Gently pull both ankles and compare the length of the legs. Are two legs unequal in length? Slightly pull both legs down with some force, as if to correct the length. Explore the vertebral bodies and their alignment. Are they in straight line? Observe the Iliac crests on both sides. Are they lined up horizontally?

Then ask her sit on heels as shown in the picture. Sit behind the patient with toes and knees touching the floor as in the picture. Ask the patient to keep the hands with fingers cross behind her head, on the occipital zone. Shove your hands through her armpits and clasp over her hands behind her head. By clasping her towards your body, lift yourself up. You may hear some cracks. In this move, the therapist straightens up and pushes the patient with his chest on the back of the patient. In this move, the thoracic upper vertebrae are readjusted.

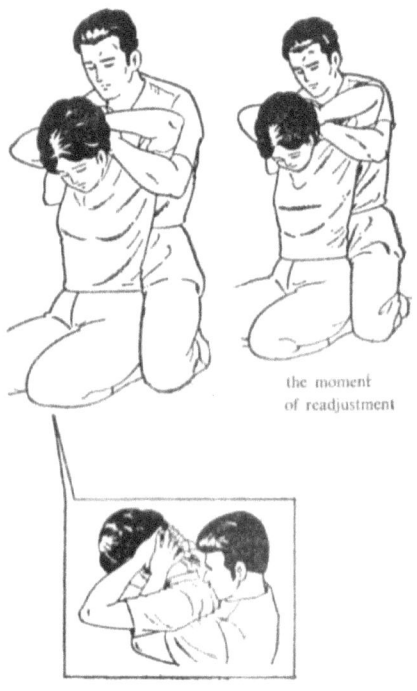
the moment of readjustment

In the next move, lower thoracic vertebrae are realigned. As in the previous move, sit behind her and hold her armpits onto your forearms as shown in the picture. With your knees pressing against her back, pull up her with your forearms twice or thrice slightly changing the position of your knees, from downwards to upwards, on her back. This maneuver will realign the lower thoracic vertebrae. Cracking sounds will attest that readjustments are made.

Japanese Yumeiho Therapy

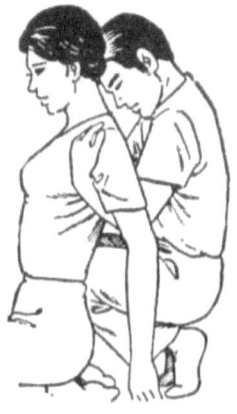
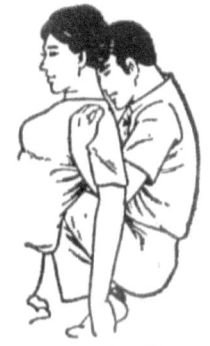

the moment of readjustment

After the thoracic vertebrae are readjusted we now focus on lumbar vertebrae. To work on the lumbar vertebrae the therapist keeps his right knee on the right femur of the patient. Ask the patient to keep her right palm/hand over left shoulder. The therapist shove his left hand under the patient's left armpit and clasp over her back of her hand. The therapist keep his right palm over right shoulder of the patient and push the right shoulder forward and pull her body backwards with your left hand. Overcome the resistance and pull & push with a jerk. This movement will swivel the spine, mainly the lumbar vertebrae. During this movement, you may hear cracks indicating the readjustments. This maneuver should be done on other side too. In this move, the therapist keeps his left knee on the left femur of the patient. She keeps her left hand over right shoulder. The therapist clasps her right shoulder with his right hand and pushes her left shoulder with his left hand.

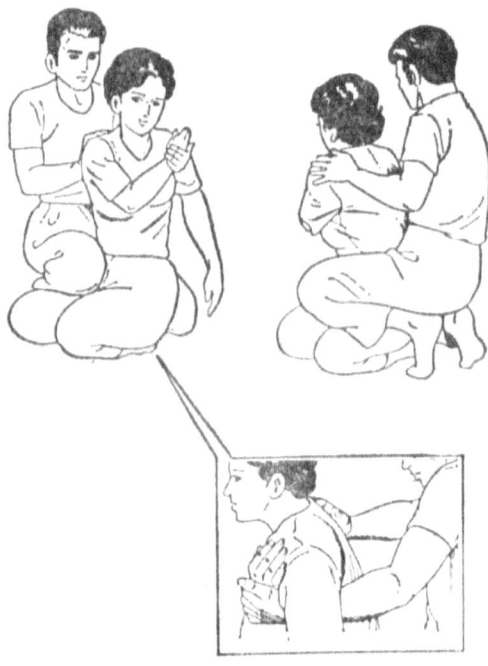

After adjusting the thoracic and lumbar vertebrae the sacrospinal muscles on the back are to be press knead. The sacroilac joint is weight bearing articulation and clinically very important. Press-kneading the sacrospinal muscles helps soften the rigid musculature from neck to hip. To press knead the upper portion of the sacrospinal musculature, the patient lies on belly and the therapist sits on the side of the patient on heels. Using his palms and fingers, the therapist press knead the area above the scapula ten times each on both sides. Alternatively, straddle the patient's hips with your knees resting on the floor. Then, knead above the shoulder blades with your thumbs 10 times each spot.

Press kneading the thoracic vertebrae follows these moves. The therapist sit across the legs of the patient, as in the previous move, and press knead along the spine on both sides ten times each. We will then proceed to readjust and invigorate the sacroiliac joint. The sacroiliac joint is one of the most important joints, whose dysfunction may cause unbearable and untreatable pain.

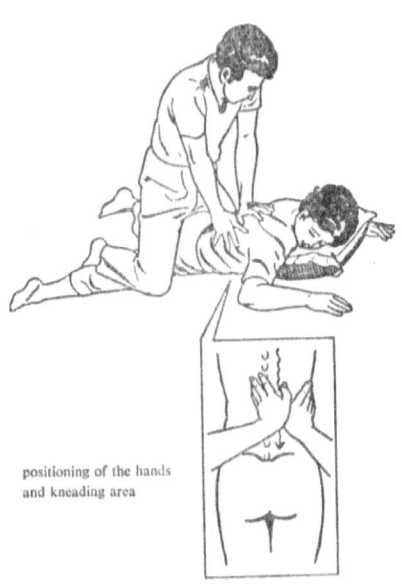

positioning of the hands and kneading area

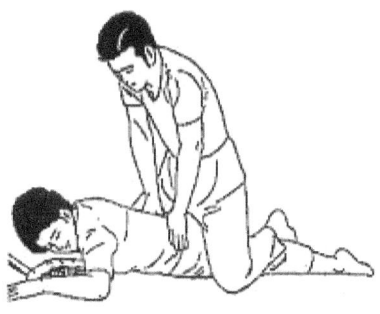

To realign the sacroiliac joint, ask her to lie on right side of the body. Let her keep the left leg slightly folded and positioned forward. Her left hand extended back. The therapist keeps his right and left knees on both sides of left leg of the patient, as shown in the picture.

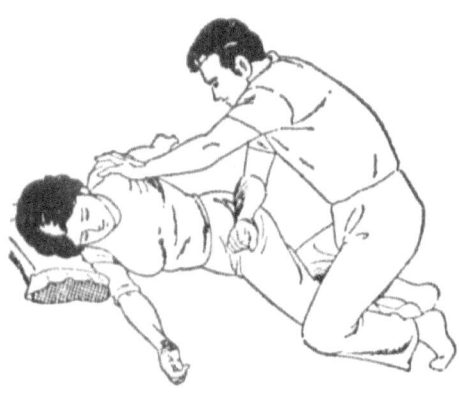

The physician keeps his right forearm on the right hip of the patient and left hand on the left shoulder of the patient. In this position, push the hip and shoulder in opposite directions to swivel the spine. This maneuver will give cracking sounds. To adjust the sacroiliac joint on the other side repeat the movement by asking her to lie on her left side and extend her right leg slightly folded and forward. The physician now keeps his left and right knees on both sides of her right leg. Then push her shoulder and hip in opposite directions to realign the sacroiliac joint.

The final step in the fundamental movement is adjusting the hip joints on both sides. Ask the patient to lie on her right side, with both hands forward. Sit at the feet of the patient on your hips. Let her keep the right leg folded and left leg straight down. Hold the left foot at ankle with your both hands and gently and suddenly pull the leg. You may feel a clasp sound. Hip joint is readjusted in this move.

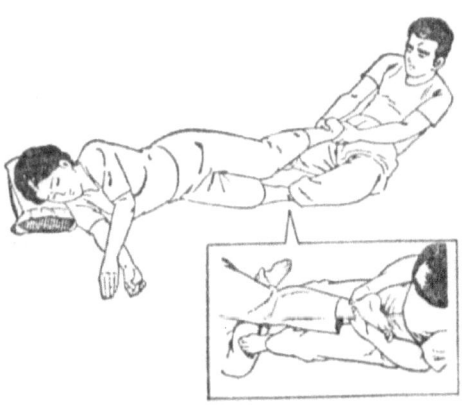

Repeat this movement on the right leg too. While readjusting the right leg, the patient lies on her left side and folds the left leg as in the picture.

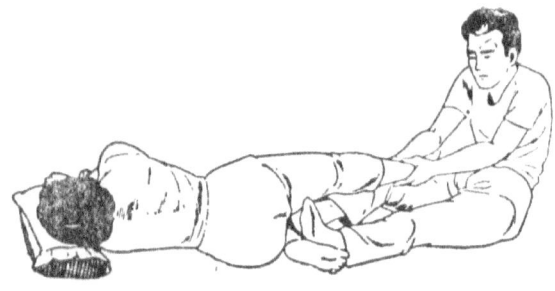

In these sixteen fundamental movements, eleven maneuvers adjust the articulations and five areas are press kneaded. Apply these maneuvers on all, who seek assistance of Yumeiho therapist. After concluding these fundamental movements, another one hundred movements selectively applied. However, you have to assess what kind of movements are required basing on the signs and symptoms.

The remaining one hundred maneuvers are grouped according to the area of application. These maneuvers are selectively applied depending on the nature of complaints. In the case of lumbago, all the movements earmarked for spine and lower limbs may be applied. When a patient complains of shoulder pain and no complaints below the waist, apply fundamental movements and those maneuvers applied on the upper limb. In the case of headache and neck pain, maneuvers on head and neck may be applied. In general well being, use all movements as prophylactic measure.

While applying these one hundred movements, the therapist may choose to divide them into several classes like those applied while patient lies down on the back, on abdomen or sitting. This categorization may reduce the trouble for the patient because all the maneuvers that are applied while lying on back may be applied in a row without changing postures frequently.

Here we see the rest of one hundred Yumeiho movements.

On Spine

1. **Pull the cervical vertebrae**: Let the patient lie on her back without a pillow. The therapist sits behind her head and holds the chins with both hands. The therapist should push the shoulders of the patient with his legs gently and pull up head with both hands. Do not use excessive force. This move will reduce strain in the neck. This move is very helpful in the spondylosis. Spondylosis is a degenerative condition of the spine and can occur at any part of the spine. This technique is similar to 'traction', the physiotherapists apply with different weighing stones. Apply this movement when you press knead the face and some points on the head. Before you pull the head with your feet kept on the shoulders of the patient, slightly press the muscles of the neck with your fingers.

Japanese Yumeiho Therapy

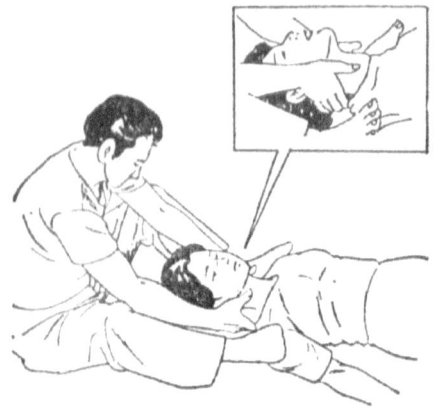

positioning of the therapist's hands and feet

2. **Flex the neck**: Let the patient lie on her belly and the therapist straddle across her body as in the picture below. Using the left thumb, the therapist press knead the trapezius muscle on the right side. Using the right thumb press knead the trapezius muscle on the left side. Press-kneading three or four times with your thumb is enough. This movement gives immense relief to the patient.

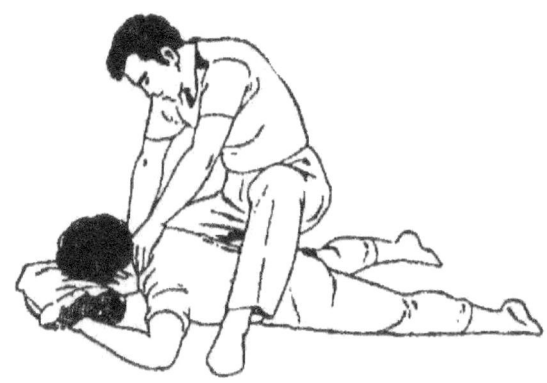

3. Later, in the same posture, press down the left shoulder and head while face is looking at left. Press the right shoulder and head while the face is looking at right. Use your right hand on the left shoulder and your left hand on the head. Just press once or twice. These moves will fix the neck bones.

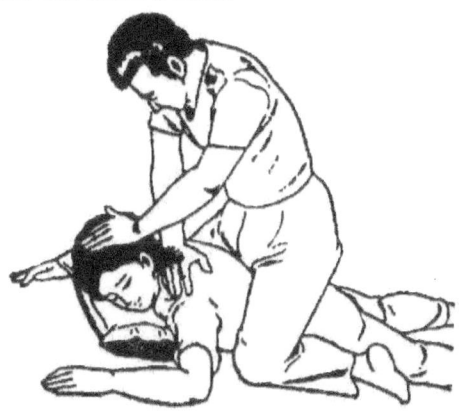

4. **Readjustment of the Neck bones**: Sit on your toes behind the patient, holding the region halfway between neck bones and thoracic vertebrae with your right thumb (your right arm should touch patient's shoulder) and the left side of her head with your left hand. While turning her head towards right or left push it suddenly towards the shoulder. The neck bones will adjust with a crack. Never use force against their hardness. Perform similar therapy on both sides of the neck.
5. **Readjust Thoracic vertebrae**: This is explained under Fundamental Movements. See the pages 42 & 43.

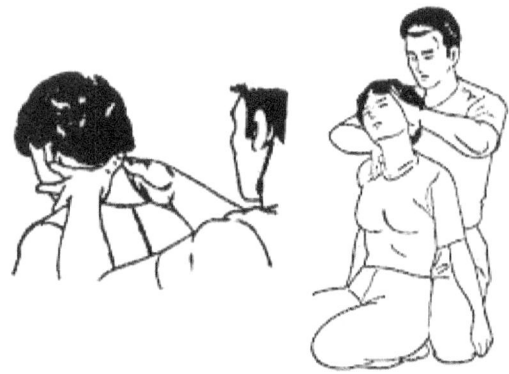

6. **Adjust the Shoulder Joints**: The patient should sit on knees and the therapist behind her. When the patient keeps her both hands on the back of the head, as shown in the picture below, the therapist hold her hands across and press. With this move her shoulders are extended. Do this movement once again.

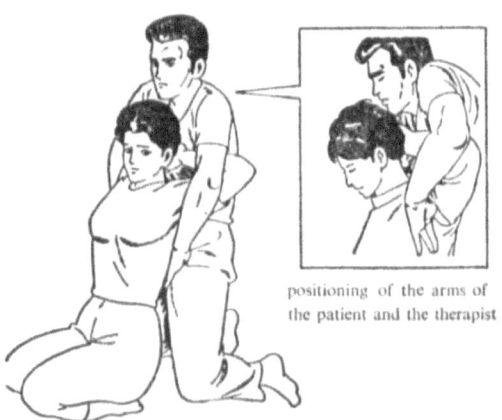

positioning of the arms of the patient and the therapist

7. **Working on Lumbar vertebrae**: This is explained under Fundamental Movements.

8. **Kneading the erector spinae with kneecaps**: Put your hands on the patient's hands softly, and slide your knees along her erector spinae on both sides from the shoulder blades down to her hips. This movement uses your bodyweight so do this movement gently. While your hands take half the bodyweight, delicately rub on her back with your knees. Try to rest your weight on five points while sliding your knees.

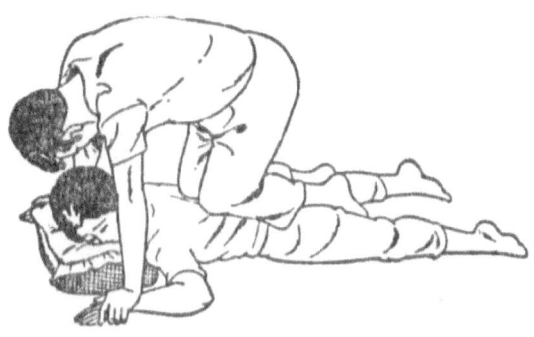

9. **Back-breaking**: First, let the patient sit on her heels and you behind her. Take her into your arms through her armpits keeping your knees against her back just above the hips. Your palms hold her shoulders. Gradually fall back as shown in the diagram and keep that pose for 3 seconds. Ensure that the patient's feet keep touching the floor firmly. In that pose, knead the region above the right and left iliac ridges with your kneecaps 5 times on both sides. Be in this posture for few seconds. Be careful while releasing the patient from your grip. The patient's body weight is hold by the therapist's kneecaps.

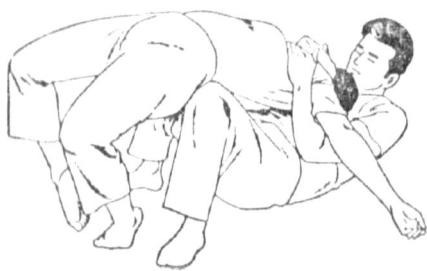

Press kneading on Spine:

1. **Press knead Trepizious**: It's a triangle-shaped wide, flat and large superficial muscle extending between back of the head to thoracic vertebrae and scapula bone. This is responsible for moving, rotating and stabilizing the scapula or shoulder blade. With your right thumb press knead the left trepezius at the neck. Use your left thumb to press knead right trepezius five times each on the neck. Later, press-knead with both hands below from the neck four or five times.

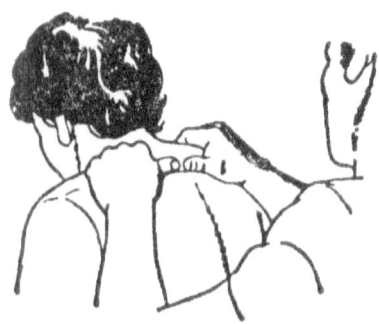

2. **Press knead Trepizious in lying posture:** While the patient lies on front, the therapist work on the trepizious

a shown in the image. Keep your knees on the floor and your feet touching the floor between the legs of the patient. Press-knead on trepizious on both sides for few moments.

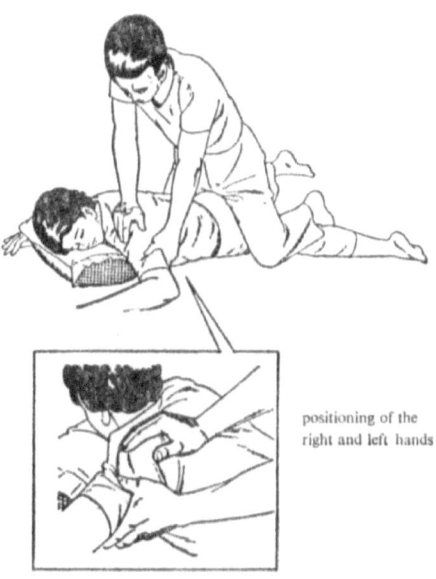

positioning of the right and left hands

3. **Press knead Sternocledo mastoid**: It's a large surface muscle originating at the sternum, breastbone, and clavicle or collar bone and inserting on to the mastoid process of the skull in the back. This muscle helps in rotation of head and flexion of neck. The therapist sits behind the patient and using his thumbs press knead this paired muscle five times each in the neck. We use pillow while sleeping to prevent this muscle from pressing the thoracic cage down that causes difficulty in breathing while sleeping.

4. **Press knead the Shoulders**: The patient sit on her knees and the therapist stand behind her. The therapist using his knees support the back of the patient and with his hands press knead her shoulders above the scapula for five times as shown in the picture.

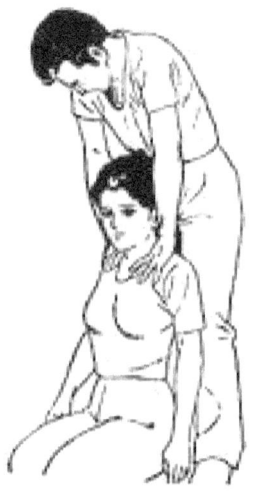

5. **Kneading the Erector spine above the shoulder blades**: This is covered under Fundamental Movements.
6. **Kneading the back**: Straddle across or sit on one side of her as shown in the picture in the next page. Using your fingers and bulb of your thumb press and knead along the spine. This move will smoothen the muscles on both sides of the spine. Keep your right palm over the left thumb and left palm over right thumb while pressing on the back.

Japanese Yumeiho Therapy

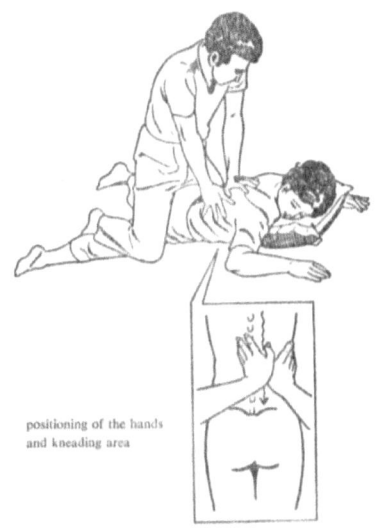

positioning of the hands and kneading area

7. **Kneading the Sacral region:** Let the patient lie on her belly, stretching out her legs. Straddle across her hips settling your knees on the floor and your toes between her legs as shown in the picture below. Then, knead 4 to 5 spots in sacral region with your thumbs, 3 times each. However, never press coccyx strongly. While doing this maneuver, let the patient's toes directing inwards not outwards.

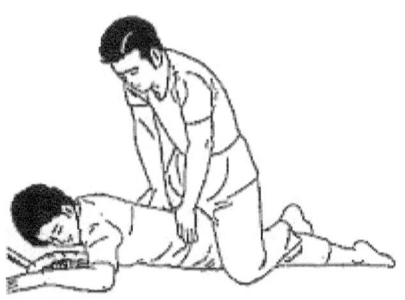

On Upper Limbs

The patient lies on back. The therapist sits on the right side of the patient to carry out these manipulations on the right arm and on the left side to deal with left arm. These movements are done on both sides i.e. on both arms. While working on right arm, the therapist uses right hand to press knead shoulder muscles and axillary region. While doing on left arm, the therapist use left arm to press knead the shoulder and axillary region. While the therapist is applying Yumeiho on left arm, let the patient turn the head towards right. Similarly, the patient turns her head towards left while the therapy is applied on her right arm.

1. **Extend the Arm**: The patient lying on the back extend the right arm upwards as shown in the picture. The therapist sits on knees on the right side of the patient and keeps his right hand on the right axilla of the patient. Hold the right elbow of the patient with your left hand and press towards floor.

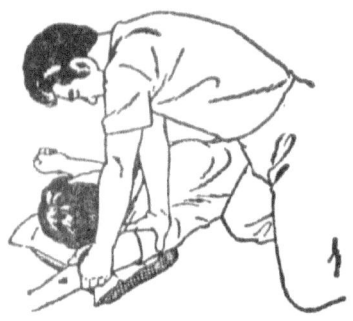

2. **Press knead axillary muscles:** With your left thumb press ten to twenty times deltoid, pectoralis and latismus dorsi muscles.

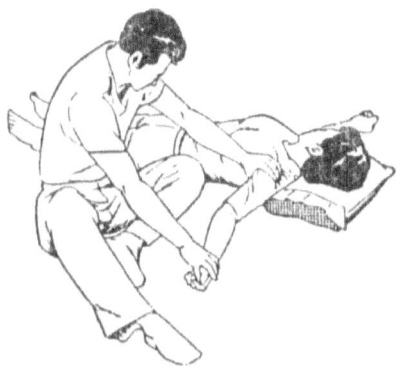

3. **Press the Shoulder:** Using your lower part of the palm above the wrist press on the shoulder muscles few times.
4. **Pull the Arm:** Keeping your right foot against the right axilla of the patient, gently pull the arm with both hands. While pulling, grasp the palm of the patient with your left hand and use your right hand to clasp over patient's hand on the back.

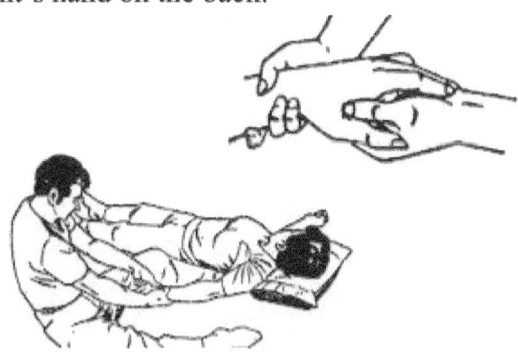

5. **Press knead Trapezius muscle**: Let the patient lie on belly. The therapist sit on knees across the patient's hips, as shown in the picture on page 55, and hold the trapezius muscle with right hand (for patient's right hand) at the shoulder and with left hand for patient's left hand. Press knead few times at the shoulder area of trepezius.
6. **Readjustment of the Elbow Joint**: Hold the patient's elbow from underneath with your left hand, and her wrist with your right hand. Then suddenly push up your left hand while pulling down the patient's hand so that the elbow is stretched. Jerk up twice.

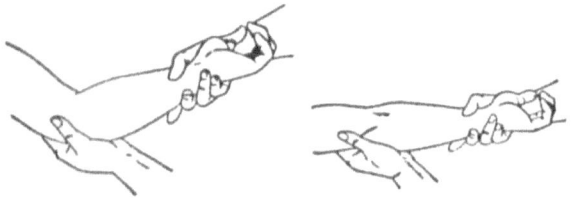

7. **Readjustment of the Wrist**: Hold the wrist with your index and middle fingers from below and keep both thumbs on the wrist. Slightly move your thumbs back and forth so that the hand of the patient moves up and down. Do it with some force suddenly so that the wrist bones are readjusted.
8. **Press knead Right Forearm**: Hold the patient's right forearm arm at the wrist with your right hand and use your left hand fingers to press knead in the area above the wrist.

9. **Press knead the Right Palm**: The therapist hold the palm of the patient by keeping his little finger of the left hand between the thumb and index finger of the right hand of the patient. Similarly, keep the little finger of the right hand between the ring finger and little finger of the patient's right hand. Use your thumbs to press the palm of the patient, particularly on the ball of the thumb and nearby area. While doing so your three fingers (ring, middle and pointing) support the hand from below.

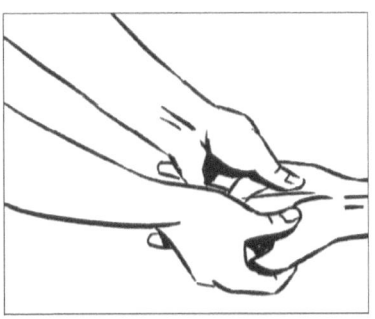

10. **Slide over Radial Nerve**: Hold the patient's right hand with your right hand as if you are shaking hands. Keep your left thumb over the forearm as if palpating the radial nerve. Then turn the right hand of the patient back and forth to slide over (with your left thumb) the radial nerve. This movement may be slightly painful. You may slightly increase pressure with left thumb. These movements will stimulate the radial nerve.

11. **Press the area between thumb and index finger**: The therapist press the area between the thumb and index

finger on the hind side of the palm. To do this movement, keep your thumb on top, as shown in the diagram, and index finger under. Then gently press the area. This may be little painful to the patient. While doing so, use your left hand to hold the patient's hand for support.

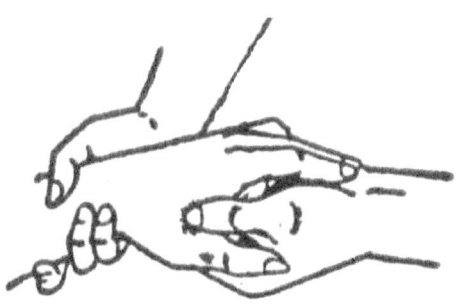

12. **Adjust the Wrist**: Let the patient extend her right hand with palm downwards. The therapist should firmly hold the wrist with fingers of both hands and press knead down up to fingers. Use your palms area for pressing of the fingers. Do this pressing of palms twice or thrice so that patient feels elated.
13. **Readjustment of Phalanges**: Hold the patient's right wrist with your left hand. Pull each finger using your fingers of right hand applying gentle pressure. All fingers may crack. Hold each finger between your middle finger and pointing finger for better grip while pulling.
14. **Extend the arms**: Sit behind the patient and take hold of both forearms as shown in the picture. Bring closer

the arms slowly as far as possible. Do not apply sudden force or jerks. See how far the arms are flexible.

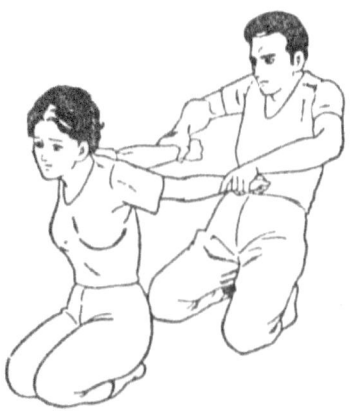

15. **Stretching of Arms backwards**: Sit behind the patient, as in the previous posture. You and she sit on folded knees. If the patient is unable to sit on folded knees, let her sit, as she likes. Then hold her shoulders with your both hands and pull back towards median line three times so that her chest is spread.

16. **Tap on the back**: Now we come to last steps on upper limbs. Clasp your fingers as shown in the picture on the next page and tap on the back vertically and horizontally twice. The line of tapping is given in the diagram. This tapping with your clasped palms will give a feeling of elation to the patient.

Japanese Yumeiho Therapy

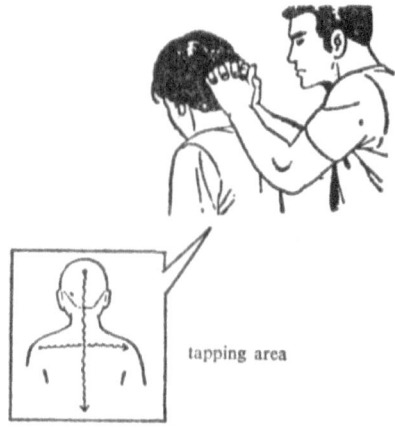

tapping area

17. **Tossing the Shoulders**: Hold the patient's shoulders with your hands as shown in the image. Then lift and release them. Repeat this lift-release exercise, five times.

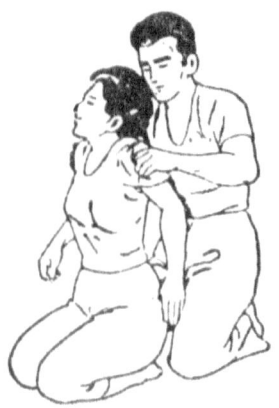

Repeat all these movements on the other arm too.

On Head & Face

Let the patient lie on back on the floor and the therapist sit behind the head of the patient, as shown in the diagram below. Use a thin cotton cloth to cover the patient's face. Palms of the therapist should not touch the skin of the patient directly. Pressing and kneading on the facial muscles is very important for a healthy mien.

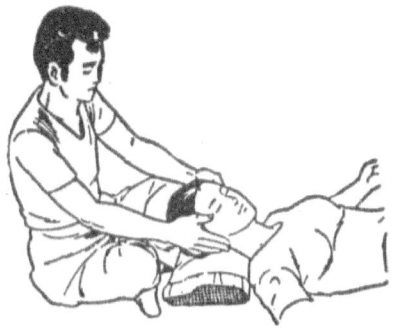

1. **Kneading the sides of the nose**: Ask her to lie on back and spread a piece of cotton cloth across her face. Rub the sides of the nose with both thumbs with mild pressure three or four times.

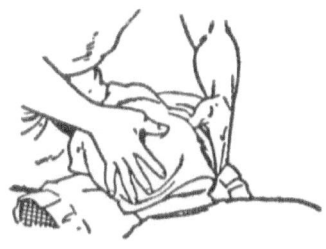

2. **Knead upper part and lower part of the temples around the eyeballs**. Delicately massage the areas around the eyes with both palms three times using your thumbs and fingers.
3. **Oppression of eyeballs**: press the eyeballs three times for three seconds each time simultaneously with your middle finger. Then slightly press the patient's cheeks with your fingers on both sides at a time.

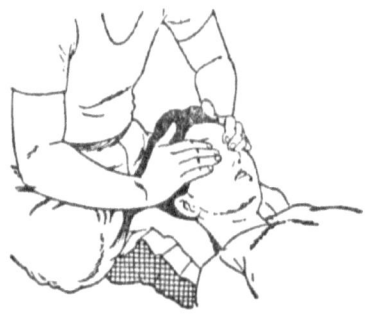

4. **Locking the face**: Clasp your fingers together across the patient's face keeping your lower part of the palms on the area of slight depression near the patient's temples on the face. And press with your palms for few moments.

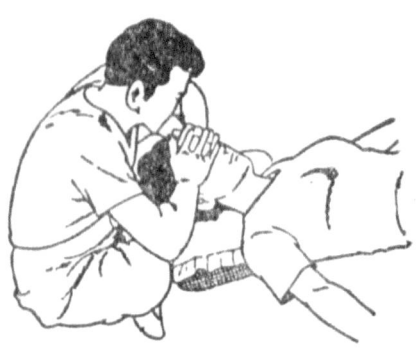

Japanese Yumeiho Therapy

5. **Pressing the midline of the head**: press with your thumbs at different points from the forehead on the line down along the medial line up to bregma on the skull.

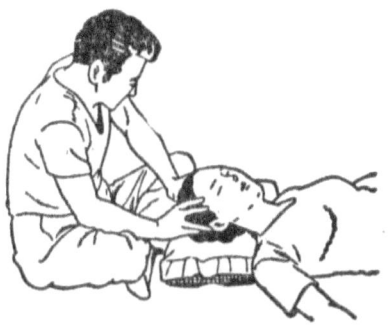

6. **Tapping on the forehead**: Clasp your both hands and slightly tap with your fingers on forehead from behind the patient. While tapping let loose the fingers so that they make sound. Do not use excessive force.

On Lower Limbs:

When the patient lies on ventral side let her keep her feet as shown in the picture. The toes of both legs face to midline.

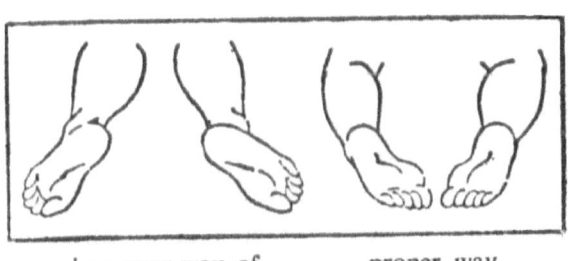

improper way of placing her toes

proper way

Japanese Yumeiho Therapy

1. **Press knead Gluteus muscle**: Let the patient lie on ventral side. Straddle across the leg of the patient and press knead the gluteus muscle twenty times with your palm and fingers, first with your thumb and later with palm.

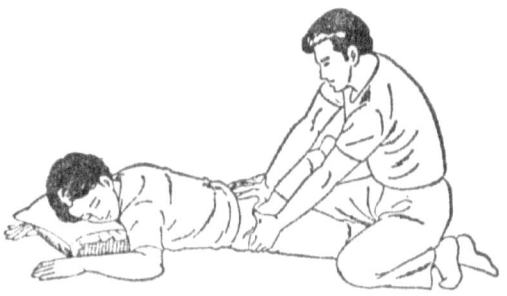

2. **Press knead Gluteal pleat**: In the similar position, press knead gluteal pleat (skin fold) ten times gently.

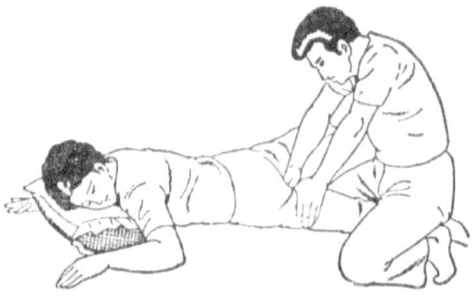

3. **Press knead Femoral Biceps**: continue to sit as in the previous session. Gently use your both thumbs to press knead from gluteal crease up to popliteal area on eight points four times each. While doing so, use your other four fingers to hold the thigh. See the diagram in the next page for appropriate areas of pressing.

Japanese Yumeiho Therapy

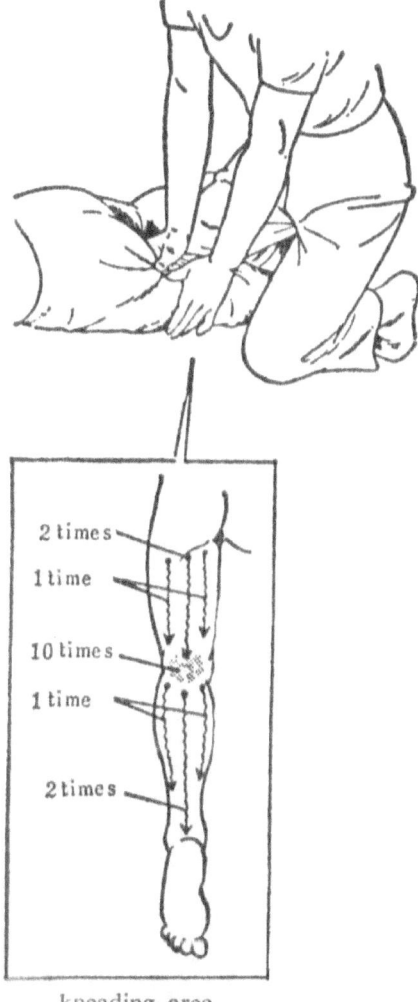

kneading area and frequency

4. **Extend the muscles of legs**: Therapist place his soles on the popliteal region, behind the knees, of the patient and take hold of feet with your fingers and slightly

press towards the hips of the patient as shown in the picture. In this posture, the therapist's body weight is born by the patient for few moments. This movement is important for knee and its muscles.

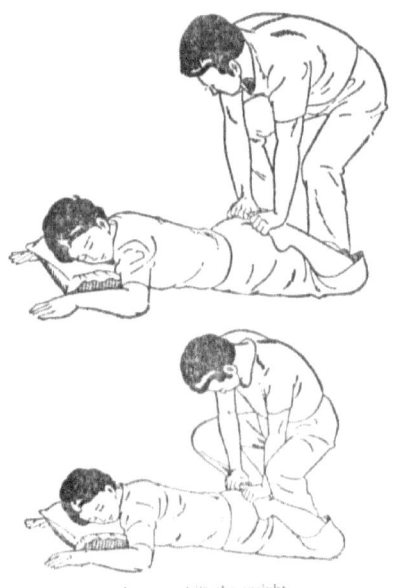

how to shift the weight

5. **Turn the left hip joint or coxal joint**: Let the patient lie on her back. Take the left knee of the patient with your right hand and ankle with your left hand as shown in the picture next page. Press the leg twice upwards and exteriorly. This will flex the knee joint. Flex and turn the hip joint and extend the knee joint two times with some force.

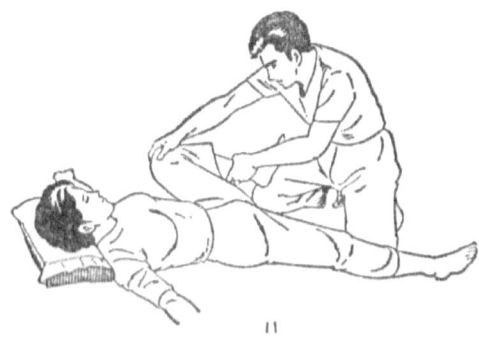

6. **Kneading the region above the right trochanter**: Let the patient lie on ventral side. Straddling her left leg, rest your knees on the floor and sit on your heels. Then thrust knead the patient's right hip with either thumb or the palm of your right hand for about 20 times.

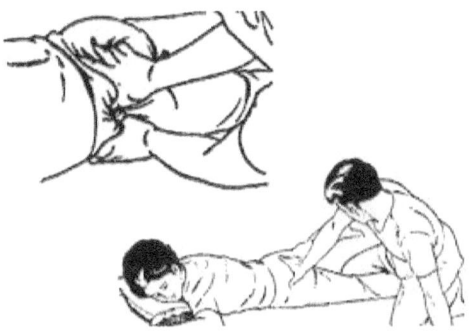

7. **Kneading the back of the knee:** Keep your knees on the floor and straddle across the leg and press knead the area behind the knee ten times with your palms and fingers.

Japanese Yumeiho Therapy

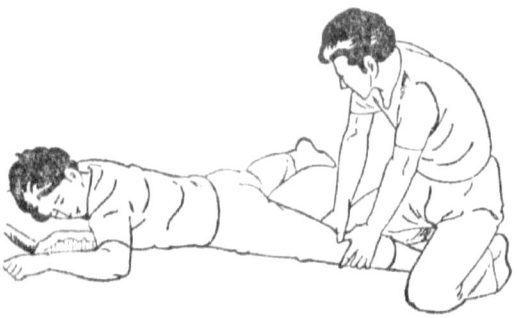

8. **Readjustment of the tarsal joints:** Let the patient lie in on ventral side as in previous move with her legs spread. Keep your knees on the floor between her legs and hold her toes of both legs with your hands and push her feet down and forward against her hips. You may hear crack.

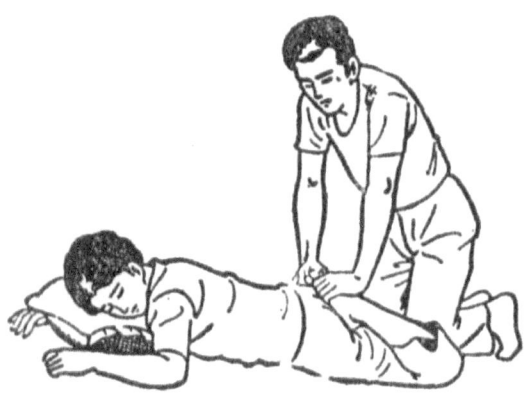

9. **Readjustment of toe phalanges**: After completing the previous move allow the patient's legs come to normal position. Take both feet into your hands and when toes

are upright, crack the toe bones of both feet at the same time.

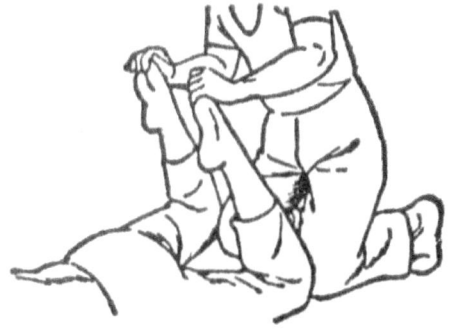

10. **Simultaneous kneading of right and left calf muscles**: Massage calf muscle tendon with your palms 10 times with your thumbs or palms.
11. **Simultaneous kneading of right and left Achilles tendons:** Using your both thumbs press across the tendons of the heel ten times.

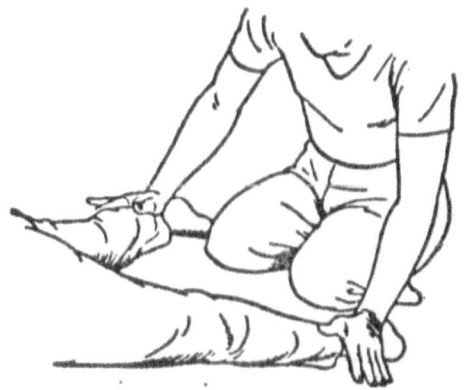

Japanese Yumeiho Therapy

12. **Press the heels:** The therapist sit between the legs of the patient and hold both heels with both hands as shown in the picture. Let the toes be pointing to median line. The therapist pushes the heels against the ground using his body weight two or three times.
13. **Press the soles:** Using thumbs of both hands, the therapist press the soles of the feet along the arch of the foot simultaneously. This reminds us of reflex points.

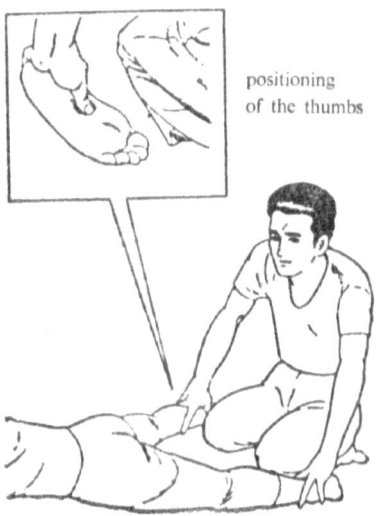

positioning of the thumbs

14. **Kneading the thigh:** Ask the patient to bend one leg inward as shown in the picture in the next page. Then straddle across the leg and press knead in three lines on six points on the quadriceps femoris muscle.

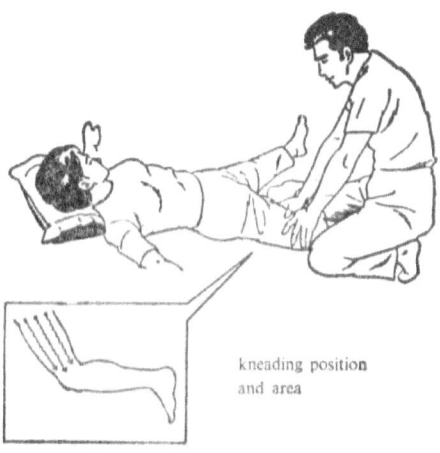

kneading position and area

15. **Extend the legs**: Now, let the patient lie on her back. Keep your both hands on her knees. Keep your left hand on her right knee and your right hand on her left knee. Widen her legs and slightly push both legs to the ground delicately. While doing this move her feet should be together.

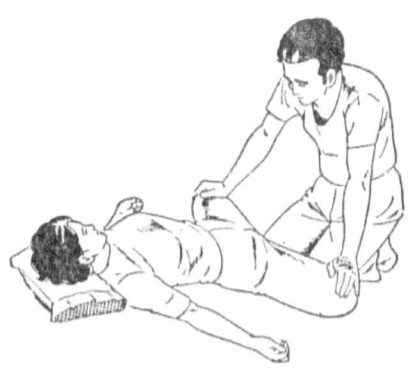

Japanese Yumeiho Therapy

16. **Fold the legs**: Take both legs at the knees into your hands, fold them to the maximum, and push against as shown in the picture.

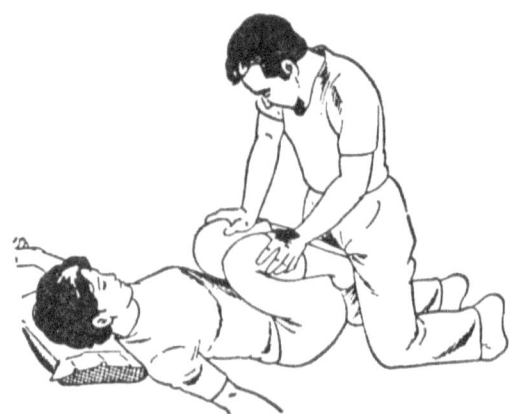

the therapist's pose in jerking

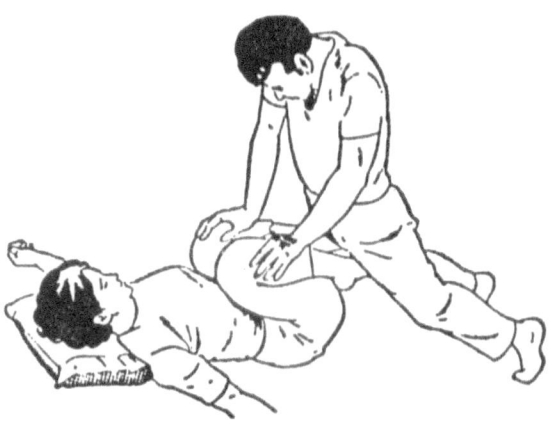

now to shift the weight

17. **Press the femur**: Sit on folded knees on one side of the patient. If you sit on left side of her, take her knee onto your both knees. Use your left thumb to press on the left side of the femur in four or five places along the lateral line.
18. **Exercise for kneecap**: Sit in the same posture on one side of her and take knee on to your both knees as in the picture. Use your thumbs and index fingers of both hands to slightly massage the area around the kneecap.

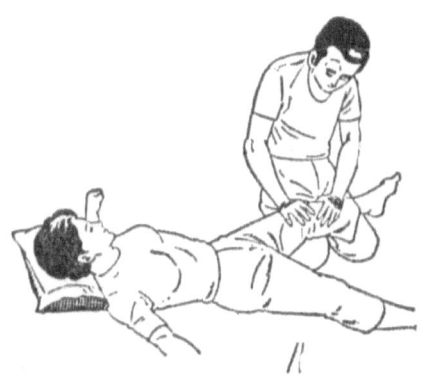

19. **Move Kneecap**: In the same posture, using your bulb of right palm, supported by left palm, press and push the bone of the knee cap upwards and downwards two or three times.
20. **Flex ankle**: The therapist continue to sit on the left side of her and keep the left leg of the patient on his knees. Hold the patient's ankle with your right hand and with your left hand hold the toes. Then with your left hand turn the heel in circular motion and press down slightly.

Turn the heel in clockwise and counterclockwise few times.

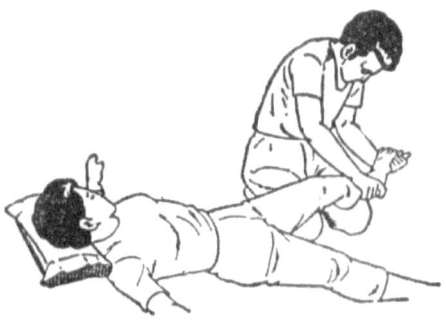

21. **Extend the heel**: In the same posture, keep the left heel of the patient into your right hand and press the feet up / towards the knee. While pushing the toes of the patient place your other forearm above the knee of the patient. This movement will extend the tendon of the heel.

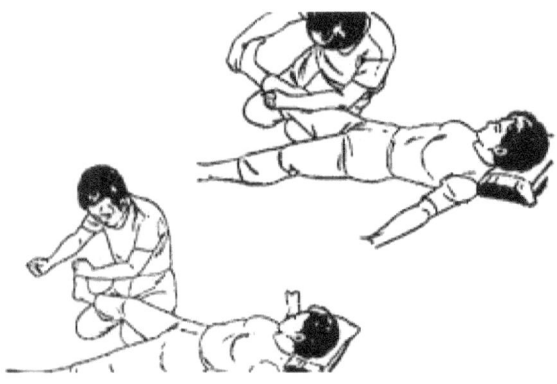

22. Beat on the left sole of the patient with your left fist twice or thrice on the heal area.

Japanese Yumeiho Therapy

23. **Readjustment of hip joints**: These moves are covered under Fundamental Movements.

Repeat all these moves on the other leg too. While repeating these movements on the other leg, your position changes and your hand movements are similar from left to right.

On Abdomen:

1. Press knead abdomen: Let the patient lie on the back and fold the knees as in the picture below. The therapist sits on one side and uses his both hands to press the abdomen from one side to the other gently. Press with bulb of palm from this side and with fingers from other side as a wave of water.

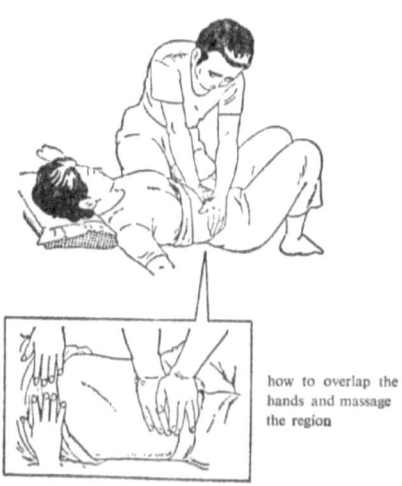

how to overlap the hands and massage the region

2. After pushing and pressing the on the abdomen over the intestines, up on your knees using your bodyweight to press over the abdomen with your both palms for few seconds.

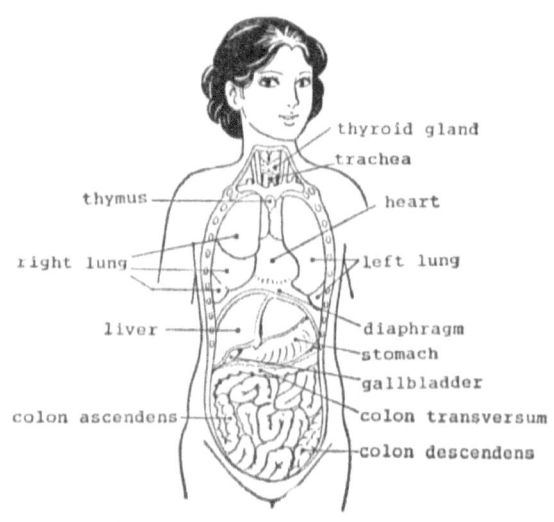

names and positions of internal organs

It is difficult to remember all postures in the beginning. Sometimes the therapist may not remember the appropriate posture of the patient too to work on. However, as you practice more and more, you remember the movements with ease. In the beginning, you may watch a video session of Yumeiho or participate in a course of Yumeiho therapy organized from time to time in various places. Find out a trained Yumeiho therapist close to your location.

Japanese Yumeiho Therapy

Muscles of the body
Ventral side

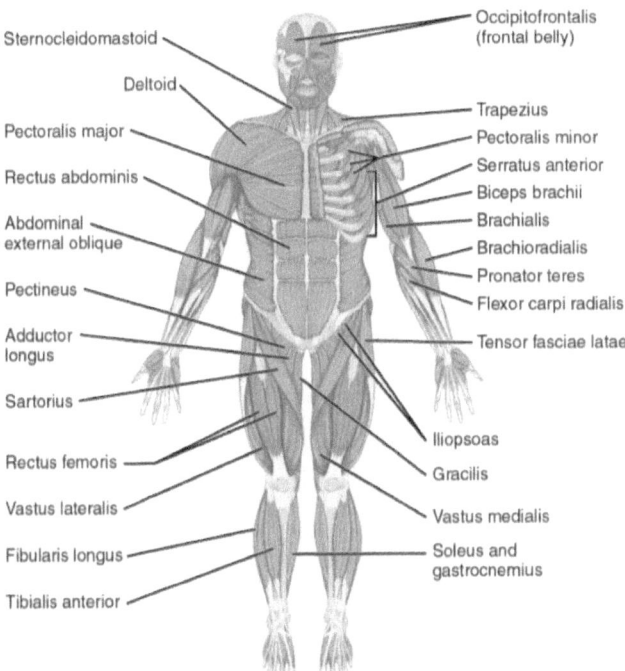

Major muscles of the body.
Right side: superficial; left side:
deep (anterior view)

Japanese Yumeiho Therapy

Muscles of the body
Dorsal side

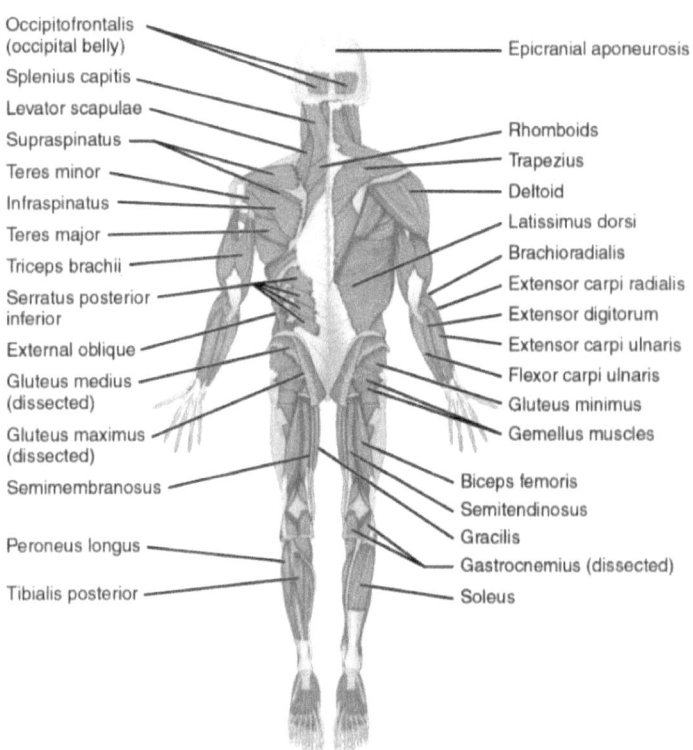

Major muscles of the body.
Right side: superficial; left side:
deep (posterior view)

Japanese Yumeiho Therapy

A note on the sequence of maneuvers: Appropriate press kneading should precede the readjustment movements on the joints. When the musculature is properly press kneaded readjusting joints is easy. Apply all the fundamental movements on all patients with some discretion of age, individual skeletal frame and flexibility of the joints. Use all techniques judiciously and carefully. There is no strict sequence of movements; however, without much asking the patient to turn sides, apply readjustment and press kneading maneuvers in a way convenient to you and the patient.

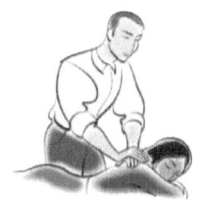

Indications and Contraindications

Yumeiho therapy is a non-invasive and drugless physical therapy. This does not mean that it is very safe. Since the healer employs various maneuvers on the patient's body, it is essential to keep in mind that it is not free of risks to the patient. Nevertheless, it is not a panacea. The therapist should keep in mind the indications and contraindications before applying Yumeiho Therapy on patients.

This therapy is very useful in men and women, who have sedentary lifestyles and hardly have time for workouts. A healthy person too can receive this treatment once a while as a preventive measure. However, few sessions of Yumeiho therapy are very beneficial in backache, low back pain (lumbago) and neck pain caused by sprain or strain, sleeplessness, fatigue, sciatica, pain in the hip joints, knees, ankles, toes and ribs; low body temperature, various headaches, stiffness or pain in the shoulders and constipation. Yumeiho also cures hypertension and hypotension. In addition, it can improve the feeling of wellbeing in diseases like muscular dystrophy, Parkinson's, cancer and autoimmune diseases like rheumatism, systemic lupus erythematosus etc. Yumeiho is effective against obesity. Mr. Saionji has treated quite a number of patients with different systemic and degenerative diseases. His data gives us general guidelines of employing Yumeiho in multiple pathologies. However, it is better to observe and record our experience and see how useful the therapy is.

Japanese Yumeiho Therapy

Yumeiho therapists across the world have documented that Yumeiho is not useful in certain diseases like parasitic infections (scabies, malaria etc.), fungal infections (mycosis, candidiasis etc.), eczema, eruptions, burns or other pathological manifestations that might spread, aggravate or cause contamination. No massages will be applied on portions of the skin, which covers area of inflammatory process (furuncles, abscesses or other purulent accumulations). No pressing and kneading will be applied in regions, which have recently undergone surgical interventions and showing incomplete or improperly healed (scarred) tissues. Do not treat patients suffering from febrile states (infectious or of any other kind), bone or osteo-articular infectious disorders (osteitis, osteomyelitis, arthritis, etc.), osteoporosis, tuberculosis of any organ, thrombophlebitis, arthritis with acute manifestation, acute cardio-circulatory disorders like angina pectoris, myocardial infarction and cardiac insufficiency.

The application of the Yumeiho therapy is also contraindicated in acute disorders of the digestive system viz. hepatic disorders, ulcerous colitis (Crohn's disease), biliary lithiasis, improperly treated (or in acute flare) gastric and duodenal ulcers. Patients suffering from renal diseases, hemorrhagic disorders (severe capillary frailty, hemophilia, treatments which require anticoagulant medication etc.), unconsolidated or insufficiently consolidated fractures and patients suffering from disk hernias accompanied by severe neurological manifestations, vertebral luxations (dislocations), any type of cancer in any stage (unless it is recommended by the oncologist), hernias of any kind are better not treated by Yumeiho therapists.

The application of Yumeiho therapy is not advisable in women during menstruation. It is better not to apply Yumeiho within at least 2 or 3 hours from the meal. Don't apply Yumeiho on children below ten years of age or senior citizens above 65 years of age. If children and old people are to be treated, the therapist should be cautious in using force, especially when tackling the neck and lumbar regions.

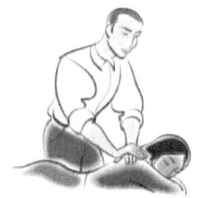

Frequently Asked Questions

1. **Can I learn Yumeiho and apply on myself?**
   You may learn Yumeiho therapy but you cannot apply it on yourself. You need another therapist to feel the experience of this therapy. Yumeiho therapist needs to train others to enjoy the fruits of therapy.

2. **Is this therapy taught in any university?**
   No, right now no university is running courses on Yumeiho therapy. However, it is taught in several Yumeiho centers across the world. Facilities are available in Japan, Poland, Rumania, United Kingdom and several other countries. The institutes imparting Yumeiho education provide certification. YouTube has multiple presentations. Browse the net to know the details about periodical courses on Yumeiho in various countries.

3. **How long it takes to learn this therapy?**
   It depends. If you are keen and a Yumeiho teacher is available, you can learn in two to three months provided you spend at least two or three hours a day. However, after the course you need more practice to acquire precision in using fingers and manipulating the joints. It is like driving, more experienced drivers avoid accidents instinctively.

4. **I am a medical doctor. Can I learn Yumeiho therapy?**
   Yes, you are a right person to learn it and practice, because you have required knowledge of anatomy, physiology and pathology. It can be advantageous and adds to your career.

Even if you belong to any paramedical professions like nurse, physiotherapist, laboratory technician etc. you still can learn it because you have some basic medical knowledge and can orientate yourself easily.

5. **I am not a medical doctor. Can I learn Yumeiho therapy?**
You can learn Yumeiho because this therapy is similar to other physical therapies and non-medical people can understand the theory of Yumeiho without an in-depth medical knowledge. However, once you start learning Yumeiho, it is advisable to read some basic medical literature to get a dimension of its application.

6. **Can I receive a testimonial about my qualification after the course?**
Yes, if you learn in a designated institute recognized by the International Institute of Preventive Medicine, Tokyo, Japan. Or else contact directly the Yumeiho centers in any country and they may be able to help you to get a testimonial.

7. **Is it legal to practice Yumeiho therapy in our country?**
It is to be explored. Usually, no government interferes in delivering services in the alternative systems of medicine; however, you may first respect the national law.

8. **I don't find a therapist in our region. Can I learn Yumeiho by reading a book and watching Youtube videos?**

No. Reading a book and watching videos of Yumeiho therapy sessions will only help you to understand the therapy and its underlying principles. To learn this great healing art you ought to seek a guru, who has profound knowledge and experience. A good teacher can give you self-confidence.

9. **I do Yoga every day. What happens if my body is handled by a Yumeiho therapist?**
No problem. Doing Yoga is not contradictory to Yumeiho therapy. If you practice Yoga regularly, the therapist can identify the degree of flexibility and symmetry in your body.

10. **I do regular aerobics and I have enough physical exercise. Is it ok, to receive Yumeihobics?**
Yumeihobics are absolutely safe in healthy people. Regular workout may not be giving enough work to all your muscles. Yumeiho can stimulate your less used muscles of your body like gluteus in the buttocks and triceps in shoulders.

11. **I suffer from Diabetes mellitus and hypertension. How about Yumeiho treatment in my case?**
Yumeiho therapy will supplement the treatment if you are on medication for diabetes and hypertension. You should not stop taking medicines to get Yumeiho therapy. However, periodically check the status and consult your physician to adjust the dosage of medicines.

12. **How to know and assess the degree of hipbone dislocation in my body?**

    Yumeiho therapist can measure the degree of your hipbone dislocation easily. However, you can assess your skeletal and muscular asymmetry by looking at wear and tear of your shoes or sandals, misaligned hipline and shoulder line. Hipline and shoulder line are to be parallel and not angling. Several ways are explained in this book to assess the asymmetry in the human body.

13. **Can a person with disability learn Yumeiho?**

    Yumeiho is about establishing physical symmetry. The therapist has to move and work a great deal. Therefore, it depends whether physically challenged person can learn this therapy. I think it is not for them.

14. **Is it ok to treat physically challenged persons with Yumeiho?**

    Yes, you can treat. However, keep in mind the degree of flexibility and bony framework of the patient while you employ certain pressure and force to press knead the muscles and readjust articulations. You have to independently assess and judge on your own to use appropriate maneuvers.

15. **Are scoliosis and kyphosis cured by Yumeiho therapy?**

    Yes, but be cautious. It is better to look at an X-ray before you start treatment. Yumeiho is a long-term process and can be an aid to correct abnormal curves of the spine. This may aid the surgery in scoliosis and kyphosis.

6. I do Yoga regularly. Do I need to do YumeihoBics?
Doing Yoga helps you to attain skeletal and muscular symmetry. Therefore, doing YumeihoBics is easier for you and adds to your physical activity. Yoga and YumeihoBics are not incompatible.

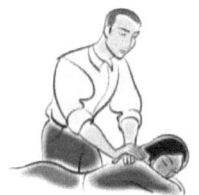

Yumeiho across the World

Since its inception, Yumeiho has been catching up the world over. Yumeiho therapists of various nationalities propagate this therapy in their localities, organize courses, run clinics and publish literature. Some Yumeiho therapists travel across the world and organize courses, teaching sessions and workshops. However, publicity and propaganda are not ethical in medicine. Any new technique or concept stands firm by virtue of its value. One of the issues of concern is increasing numbers of non-medical professionals into Yumeiho. Although this therapy can be learnt by anyone, some basic knowledge of anatomy and physiology is essential to appreciate and practice this therapy. I do not discourage persons from non-medical fields to learn Yumeiho, however, the Yumeiho centers should make the courses of long duration and include more theory in syllabus.

Originating from Japan, Yumeiho is now a popular word in Europe, South America, North America and Africa too. The first comprehensive textbook of Yumeiho appeared in 1989, which was subsequently translated into 26 languages and printed in over 20 countries. Many newspapers and journals have published articles on Yumeiho therapy. *The Japan Times* in 1989, *Passport to the New World* in 1994, *La Revuo Orienta* (monthly journal in Esperanto published from Tokyo) in 1996 have given good coverage for Yumeiho. Several TV programs have popularized the therapy. In India, the TV7, dedicated to health programs, have broadcast a 30-minute program on Yumeiho many times.

Yumeiho therapy is now popular in 73 countries. Between 1989 and 2004, Saionji travelled in 40 countries to popularize Yumeiho therapy and trained thousands of practitioners. From 1990 to 2000, the Central Military Aviation Hospital in Moscow in Russia has conducted elaborate research on Yumeiho therapy. Many of the East European nations (Hungary, Romania, Poland and Ukraine) and Baltic States (Latvia, Lithuania) have active Yumeiho centers.

With the advent of Internet several WebPages dedicated to Yumeiho appeared. Facilities were established in several European nations to study and teach Yumeiho. A wave of interest is sweeping across Poland, Germany, France, Hungary, Estonia and many nations. Literature appeared on Yumeiho in different languages. On Facebook and other social media Yumeiho therapists exchange updates, information about their experience. Courses are organized worldwide including many English speaking countries. After the demise of Masayuki Saionji, the Yumeiho center in Tokyo is continuing its academic and administrative functions.

The word Yumeiho on a browser can yield you hundreds of thousands of search results. www.yumeiho.eu website will give you details of the European organization of the Yumeiho therapists, headquartered in Poland. In

Romania, the Romanian Yumeiho Therapists Organization runs courses and healing centers in Bucharest. Several centers in US, UK and Central and South America organize periodical courses. Several ebooks are published on Yumeiho in dominant languages. However, regular university courses are not available. It is slowly spreading because it needs person to person contact in teaching and treatment. It is difficult, if not impossible. to learn Yumeiho by reading a book.

Many of its principles and techniques are already in use in physiotherapy, osteopathy, yoga, reflex therapy and other alternative healing practices. Yumeiho is catching up and going to stay along with other healing arts in the world of medical pluralism. As it has drawn much from the oriental therapies, it is a mosaic of oriental therapies.

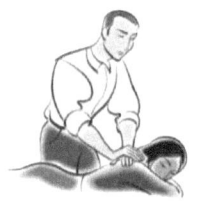

YUMEIHO BICS

Yumeiho therapy was originally designed for a trained therapist to handle patients and self-application is not possible. However, YumeihoBics (Yumeiho exercises) can be practiced at home to keep your body fit and to seek relief from minor but frequent and unpleasant troubles like pain and stiffness in hips and shoulders, irritation, dullness, sleeplessness, anxiety etc.

Aerobics is a form of rhythmic physical exercises. YumeihoBics comprises of 48 different physical movements that can be performed in few minutes. A therapist renders Yumeiho therapy, while YumeihoBics are to be practiced everyday by an individual who wants to keep his or her musculo-skeletal system in shape. As prevalence of occupational diseases is more in these days, umpteen number of people suffering from backache, lumbago, spondylitis, spondylosis, sciatica, shoulder pain, lethargy and other health problems, which are mostly caused by busy life, need to be addressed from the point of view of Yumeiho therapy. Yumeiho therapists are available in limited places across the world. Therefore, Dr Saionji has devised a set of aerobics that keep the joints and muscles in place and with right tone. These simple aerobics can be learnt in minutes and can be practiced everyday at home. These exercises will refresh the body and give a feel of Yumeiho therapy.

There are 48 movements in the YumeihoBics. Each movement needs just 5 seconds. You don't need a special place to do these aerobics. You can do in your bedroom or drawing room in the evening or morning. By doing the movements of YumeihoBics your joints will almost get back to natural position and try to make your spine erect.

While doing these exercises, sometimes you may hear cracking sounds from the joints. Each joint may crack only once and in ensuing moves the joint may not crack. Wear cottons or any comfortable dress, which do not restrict the movements. Skintight costumes are not appropriate for these aerobics.

Standing pose

1. **Re-accommodation of shoulder joints**: extend the feet equal to the width of shoulder and raise both the shoulders at once. If the flexibility is good, you hear a cracking sound. Do it for 3 to 5 times.

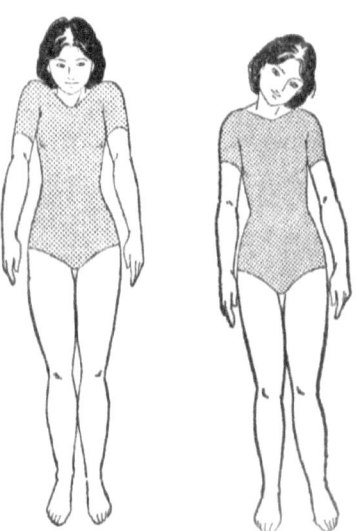

Japanese Yumeiho Therapy

2. **Adjustment of cervical (neck) vertebrae**: raise the left shoulder and simultaneously bend the head to left. Do it for few times on both sides. If you hear cracking sound the flexibility is good

3. **Stretching and flexing of neck muscles**: bend the head rightwards and lift the right shoulder up as if trying to touch the right ear with right shoulder. While tilting the head towards right keep the right arm over the left ear by arching over the head. Do similarly on the other side too.

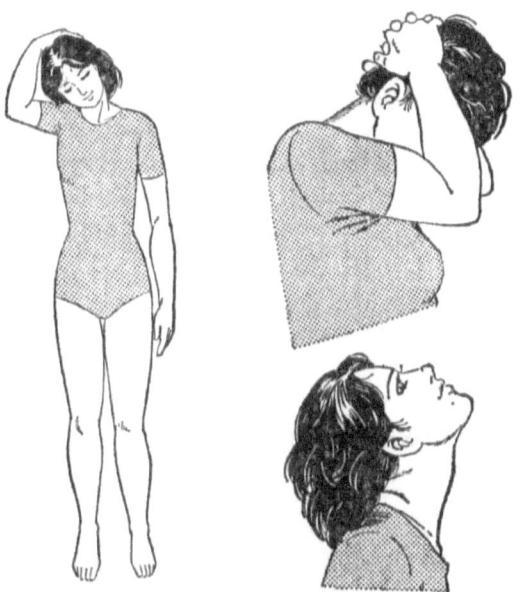

4. **Stretch neck muscles**: Bend the head forwards while both hands are pressing the head from occipital region, i.e. back of the head. Similarly lift the face backwards

to stretch the muscles of the neck as shown in the picture above.

5. Turn the head towards right side as far as possible and towards left side too. This movement will improve the flexibility and keep up the tone of the neck muscles.

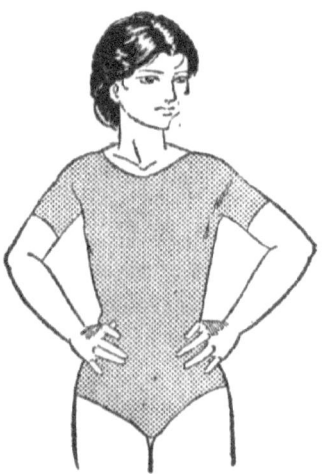

6. **Stretch and readjust the shoulder joints**: Extend both hands forward and flex with tight fist as shown in the picture. Later, swing both hands backwards and forwards few times. If you hear a crackling sound, the flexibility is excellent.

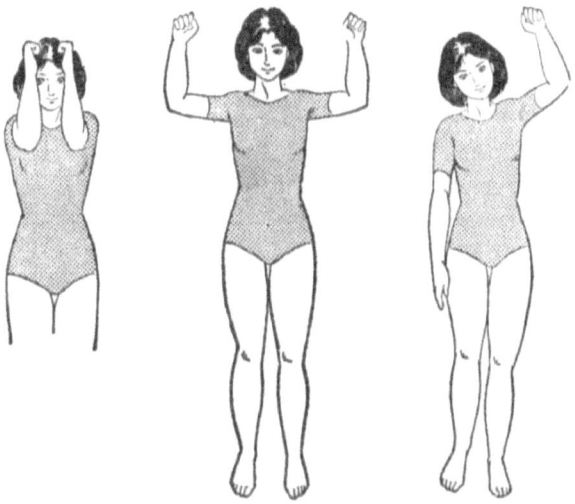

7. **Exercise the shoulder joints**: Straighten the left hand and turn it in circles first in clockwise and later in anticlockwise as shown in the third picture above. Do it with right hand too.

8. **Stretching and readjusting shoulder joints**: Take both hands towards behind and hold both together for a while, as shown in the picture in the next diagram.

9. Then catch and hold with fingers of both hands, one hand from up and the other from below. If you hear crackling sound the flexibility is good. Do similar move in opposite direction, i.e. clasp the fingers of both hand with right arm stretched from below and left from above the shoulder. If you are not able to clasp or touch the fingers behind you, practice every day.

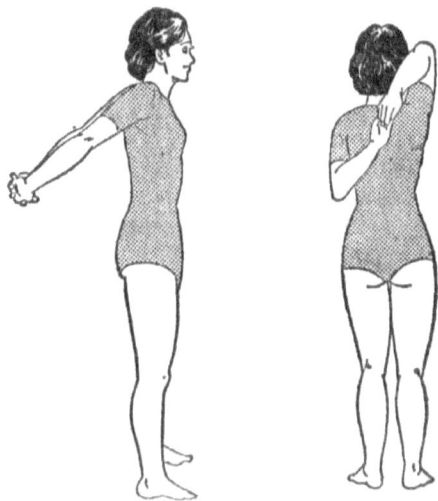

10. **Adjusting elbow joints**: Hold the right elbow with left hand and lift it upwards. Then, suddenly deliver a jerk. Do the same with right hand. If you hear cracking sound the flexibility is good.

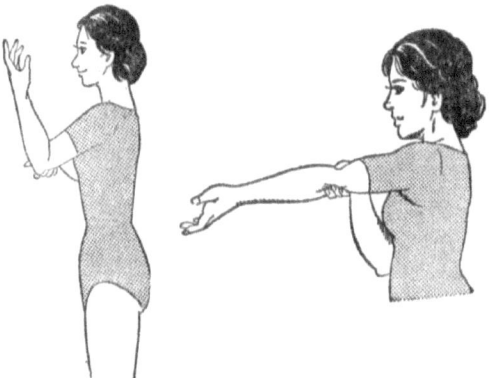

11. **Stretch forearms**: Turn the left hand slightly lateral and palm upwards and hold the fingers of left hand with

right hand and flex the fingers down. The forearm is stretched while both hands are horizontal. Repeat the same exercise with right hand.

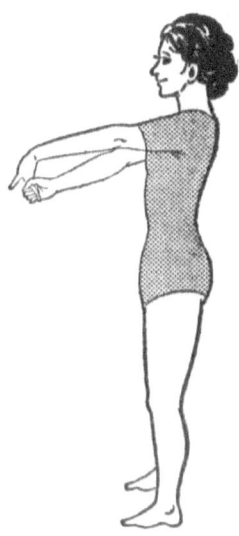

12. **Readjust wrists**: Hold the left wrist with right hand and swing it with some force. Do it with right hand too. If the flexibility is good you will hear cracking or popping sound.

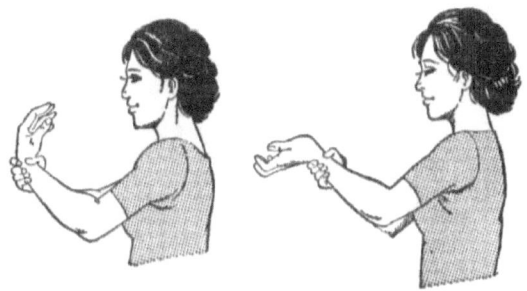

13. **Readjustment of finger joints**: Take each finger of the right hand, one by one, between the middle finger and pointing finger and tug it. Do similarly with the fingers of left hand. You will hear some cracking or snapping sounds and if no sounds are heard the flexibility is bad.

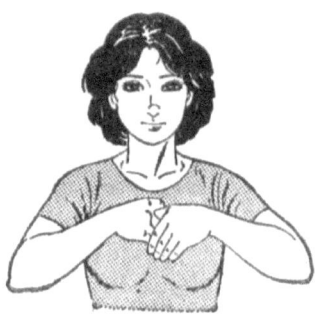

14. **Exercise for fingers**: Lift both hands and distend the fingers. Vigorously shake the hands.

15. Lift both hands up, close the fists and release them.

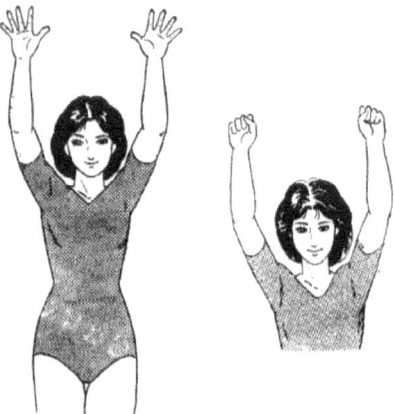

16. **Stretch the arms**: Cross the fingers of both arms in front of you while both palms are outward. Stretch the arms upwards to stretch the internal parts of the arms.

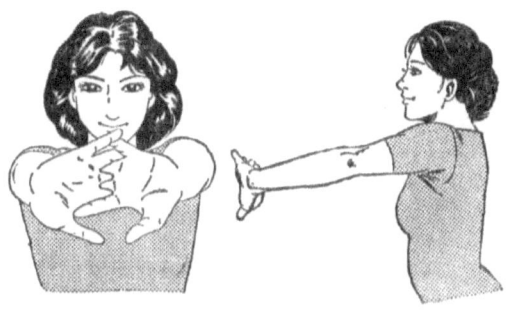

17. **Stretching and readjusting the upper sides of the trunk and shoulder joints**: Hold the left elbow with right hand behind the head and bend towards right to stretch. Repeat it by holding right elbow with left hand bend towards left. See if you hear any crackling sounds.

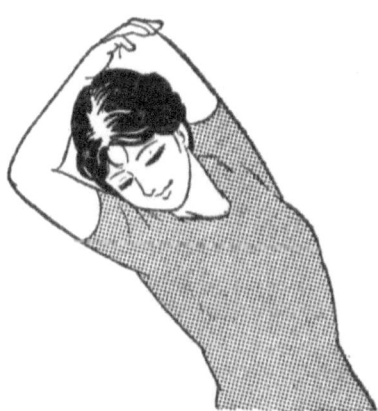

18. **Adjusting lumbar joints**: While standing on both legs, swing both hands side to side without moving your feet.

Next, hold both hands together and move the left leg towards behind the right leg. Then shift the bodyweight towards hind leg.

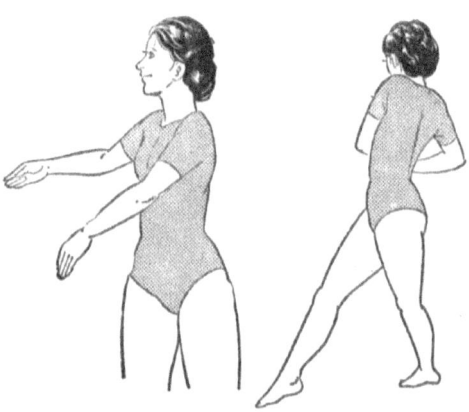

19. **Stretching the Back of the Legs**: spread the feet apart to shoulder width and stoop down as much as possible until the hands touch the floor. While doing this movement, do not bend the knees. Next, stand up and bend the body backwards.

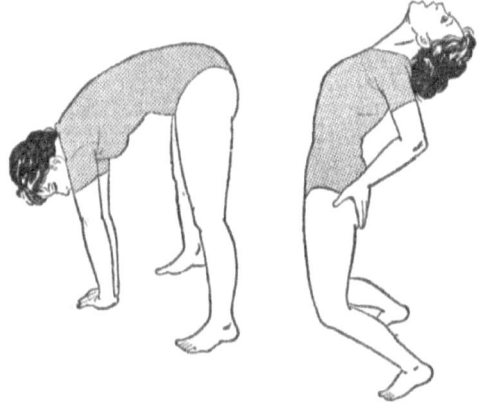

20. **Knee Joint Exercises**: Spread your feet apart beyond the shoulder width, hold your knee joints with your hands and then jostle them up and down.

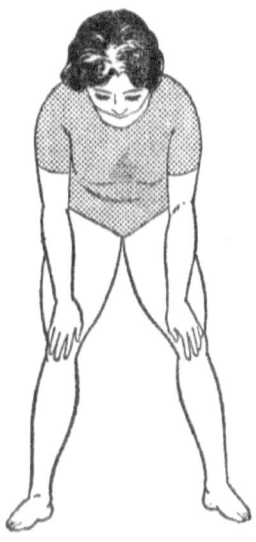

21. **Stretching the Hip Joints**: Spread your legs beyond the shoulder width as shown in the next picture, and then squat down as lower as possible. At this moment, try to straighten up your back and at the same time you do not tumble down. Push open your knees as wide as possible with your hands. If your hips come down far lower than the level of your knees, the flexibility of your hip joints is excellent. Doing it every day will gradually increase the flexibility of hip joints.

Japanese Yumeiho Therapy

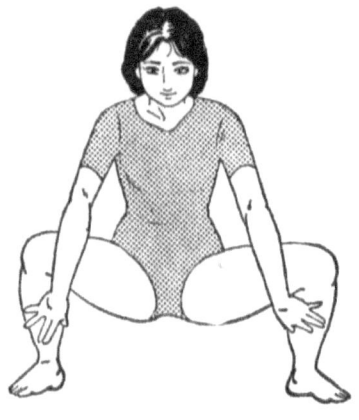

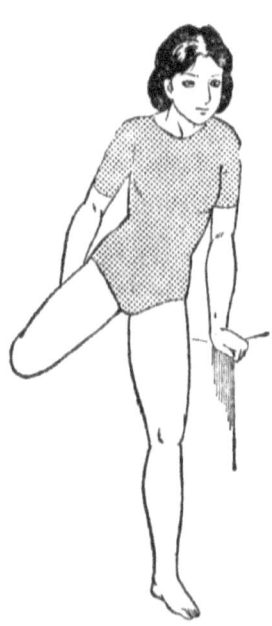

22. **Stretching the back of legs and readjustment of Hip joints**: Stand on your left leg and hold your right ankle with right hand. You may support your body keeping you left hand on a desk. Stretch the back of the legs by bending forwards. You will hear a crack if the hip joints are flexible. Do similar move using your left leg and left hand.

23. **Stretching the back of Legs**: Spread your feet wider than the shoulder width and put your hands on your knees. Slightly flex the right leg while the straightening the left leg. Press the left knee with your left hand to stretch it out. Similarly do on the other side. Next, spread the legs as far as possible and stretch them one after the other. While doing these moves try to keep your upper part of the body straight. Every time, squat as low as possible so as to take the hips closer to the ground and your hands on the extended leg as in the picture.

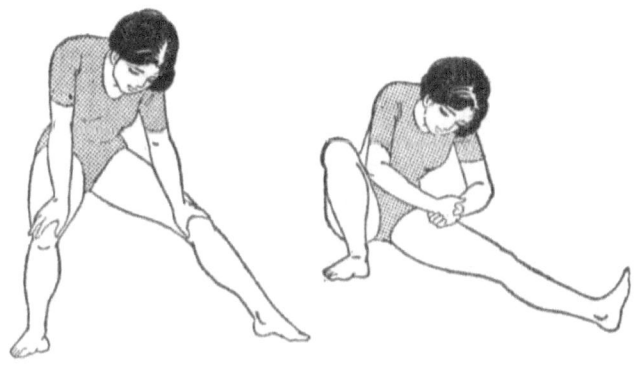

24. **Readjustment of Knee Joint and Ankle**: Stand on your right leg and lift the left leg a little. Relax your knee and give a slight jerk with force. Do this three times. You may support your body with your left hand to a wall or table. Repeat these moves with other leg.

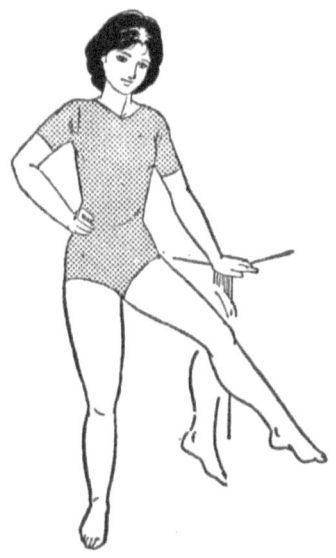

25. **Readjustment of Toes**: Place your body weight mostly on your right leg, turn the toes of your left foot inwardly and press them against the floor. Do similar exercise with left foot also. Many of the ten joints will crack.

26. **Standing on Toes**: Move your heels up and down four times, allowing your toes of both legs bear the weight of the body for some moments. See the ensuing diagrams.

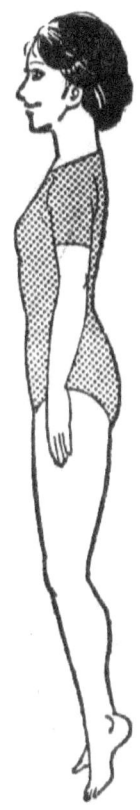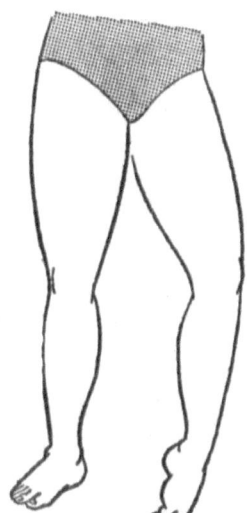

Sitting posture

27. **Stretching Hip Joints and Thighs**: Spread your feet apart as wide as possible; put your hands on the floor to support your body. Then move your whole body up and down repeatedly for some time so that the legs are well

stretched. Gradually after many days, the hips may touch the floor and you may stretch your legs 180 degrees apart. In the same posture, twist your body to the left. While keeping your body twisted, spread your feet further to the full extent, and repeat it on the opposite side.

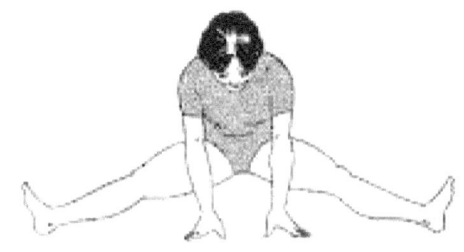

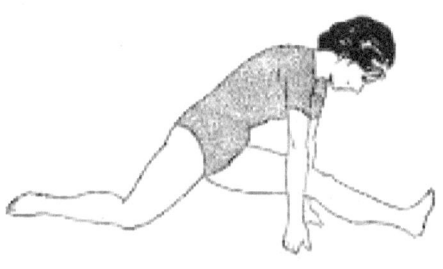

28. Sit down on the floor with legs straight and spread. Keep your hands on the ankle and lean to the floor. If your chest and forehead could touch the ground without bending the legs at knee, the inner sides of the legs and the erector muscle in the back will stretch to the

maximum possible. In the same posture, twist your body to the left, hold the toes or ankle of your left foot with your right hand. If this is difficult to accomplish, bring your hand as close as possible to the toes, trying to keep your chest on the leg. Repeat it on the other side.

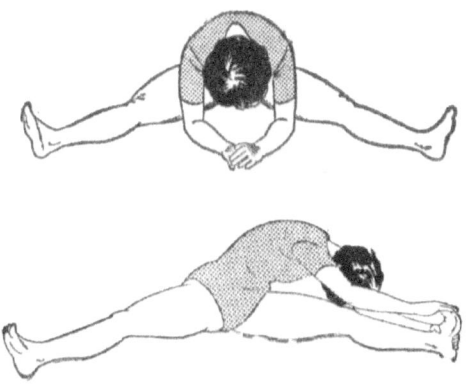

29. Sit on the floor and fold your right leg a little. Place your left leg on your right thigh. Then pull the left ankle closer to the groin and later push down your left knee with your left hand to the ground. If the knee touches the floor, the flexibility is good. Next, straighten your right leg, keep the left ankle on the right knee and hold it, as shown in the diagram, with right hand at fingers. Use your left hand to hold left ankle and slowly rotate the left foot. Repeat it on the other side too. The circular movements of the ankle will invigorate the area.

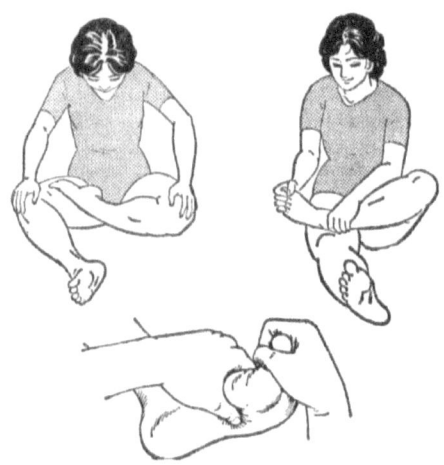

30. Put the soles of your feet together as close as possible, as show in the next picture, close to groin area. Then push down your knees with both hands to full extent. If your knees touch the floor flatly, with heels touching groin, the flexibility of the hip joints is excellent. Later, still sitting in the same posture, hold your toes with both hands and bend forward.

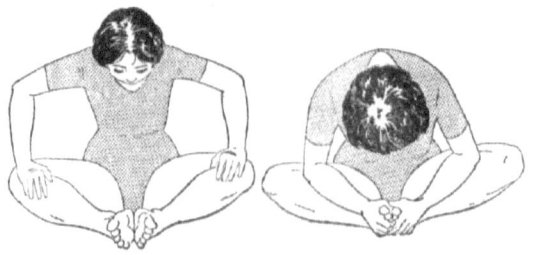

31. **Readjustment of the Vertebra**: Sit on the floor and straighten your left leg. Bring your right leg over and across your left leg and place the sole of your right foot flat on the floor. Hold the lateral side of you right knee

with your left forearm, as shown in the picture. Then twist your trunk and head to the right as far as possible. While doing so, be erect and use your right hand for support. If you hear several sounds, the flexibility is good.

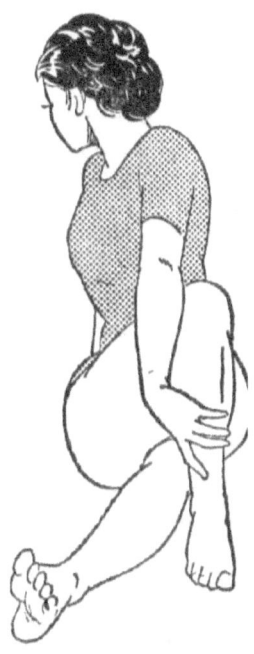

32. **Stretching the Erector spine muscles and back of the Legs**: Sit on the floor and stretch out both legs in front of you with toes upward. Straighten the knees, hold the toes with your hands, and try to bring your abdomen and chest closer to thighs.

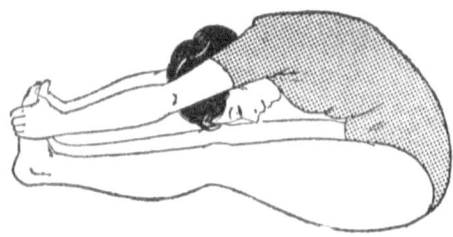

Recumbent position

33. **Stretching the Front of Trunk**: Lie down on the floor in prone position with palms on the floor alongside your body as in the diagram. Then, without moving the legs, lift your head and trunk by pushing against ground with your palms, i.e. raise your upper part of the body like a snake.

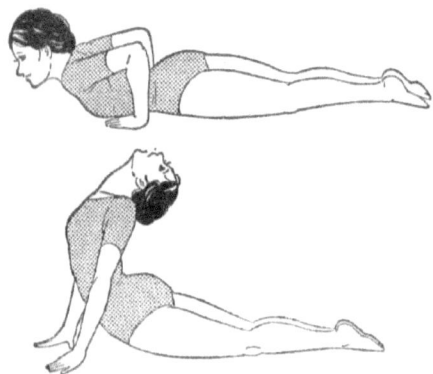

34. **Stretching of muscles in Arms, Chest, Abdomen and Front of Legs**: Rest on the floor in prone position. Hold and pull your toes with your hands so that your

back is bent like a bow. Put your knees close together and then keep the pose for a while. If you can support your body on your abdomen alone with your chest and thighs off the floor, the flexibility of your muscles in upper region of your body is excellent.

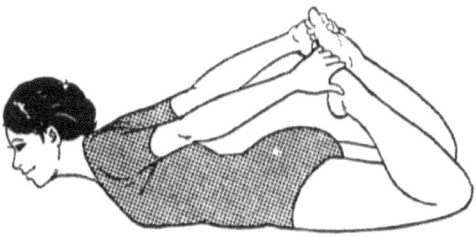

35. **Kneading the Ankles**: Sit on your heels and then twist your hips horizontally. Make sure that your heels and hips touching.

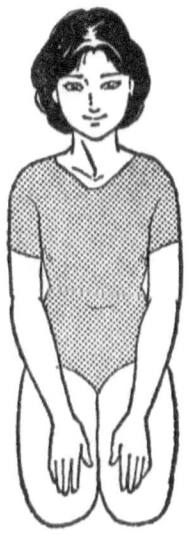

36. **Stretching the front of body and thighs**: Sit on the heels and separate them to allow your hips to drop and touch the floor. Lean back until your head touches the floor. Support your body with the elbows to make it possible without overstretching yourself. If your back touches the floor and your knees remain close together as you lean back, the flexibility is good.

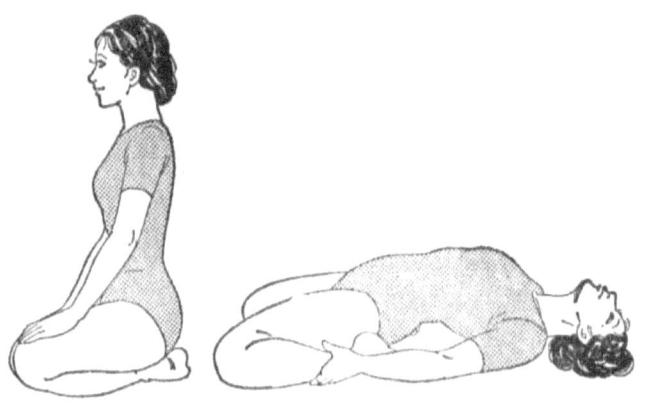

37. **Twisting the Erector and Gluteus maximus muscles and readjustment of Hipbones and Sacroiliac Joint**: To get ready for this exercise, lie on the floor on your back and extend both hands sideways. Then flex the knees and sweep them side to side as shown in the diagram. Then straighten the legs. Lift the left leg, without bending at knees, a 90 degree angle up and let it fall to left side onto the right leg. Move the right arm towards left, while quickly turning your head to the left,

so that your trunk is twisted. During the twist, left hand must be flat on the floor and shoulders should be touching the floor. These movements on the both sides show the flexibility of hip.

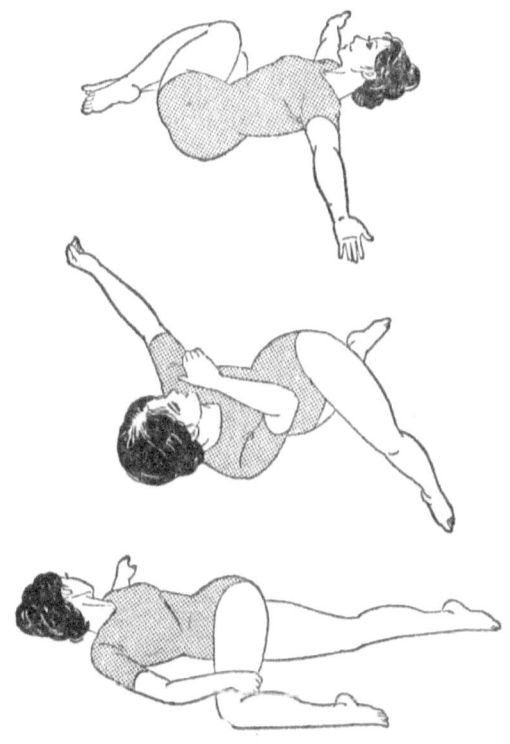

38. **Stretching the Back**: Lie down on your back and fold the legs towards the chest and hold the legs with both hands folded, as shown in the next diagram. Slowly pull the knees as close as possible to your chest. Try to put your forehead between the knees.

39. **Readjustment of Ribs**: Sit on the floor, fold your hands over your legs below the knee and roll back with force. Pull your knees towards your chest while your hips and lower back come off the floor. Keep your head forward to prevent it from hitting the floor. Then you may hear several chest bones cracking.

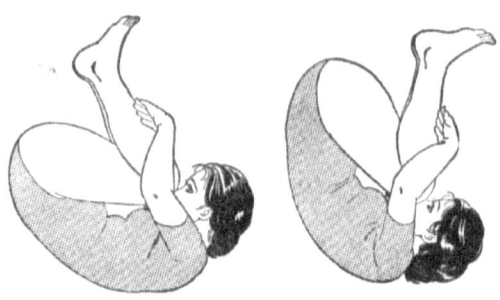

40. **Stretching the Trunk and Back of the Legs**: Lie down on the floor with both hands alongside your body and palms downwards. Raise the legs straight up without bending at the knees. Later, bend them over your head until your toes touch the floor. Then push out your heels. If the toes touch the floor, the flexibility is excellent.

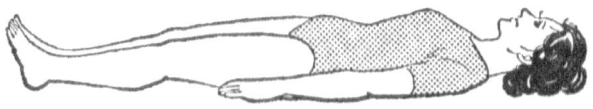

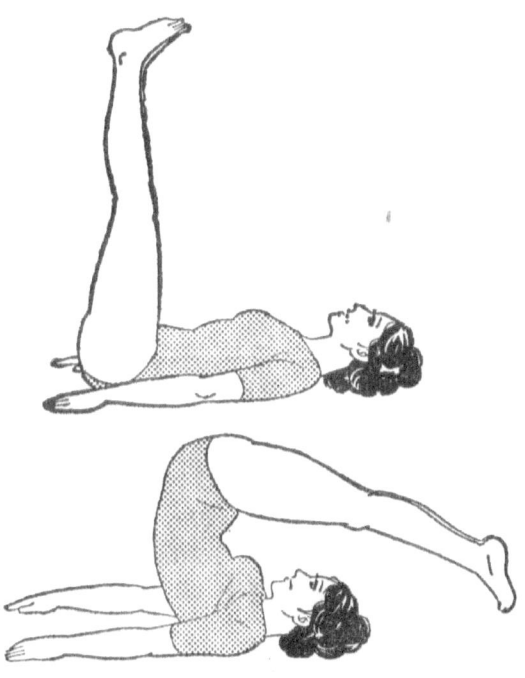

41. **Readjustment of the Upper Chest Bones**: Lie down on the floor with your knees up and feet flat on the floor. Fold your hands behind your head and pull it so that your head is lifted. Bring your elbows closer to your face and extend them to the sides while maintaining head in forward position. During the exercise, several ribs may crack. Now you are reaching the last part of the YumeihoBics. After few steps, you relax for a while to start your energetic day.

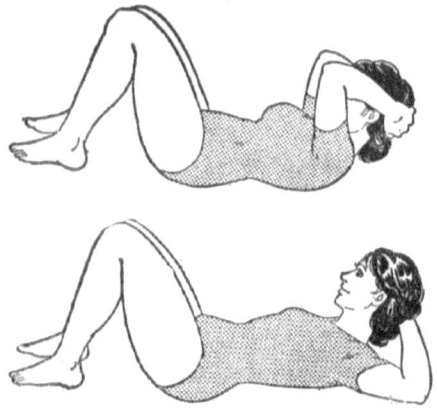

42. **Readjustment of Hip bones**: Lie down on the back with your knees up and you support your head with your hands. Then, forcefully stretch-out the knees sideways. Repeat it several times and you may hear cracking sound.

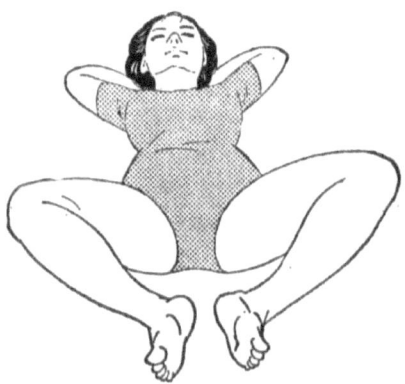

43. **Readjustment of the Tarsal Joints**: Lie down on your back with right knee up and keeping the left ankle on the right thigh. Then suddenly push down your left leg

to the floor without removing the ankle from the thigh. Do the similar move on the other side.

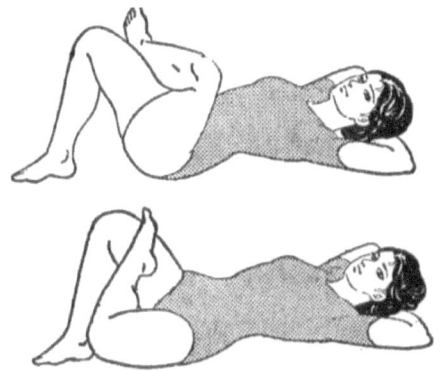

44. **Readjustment of Knee Joint**: Lie down on your back and place your hands close to your body. Relax your left knee, raise your left leg a little, and deliver a kick with full strength so that the knee is stretched and readjusted. If both knees crack, the flexibility is good.

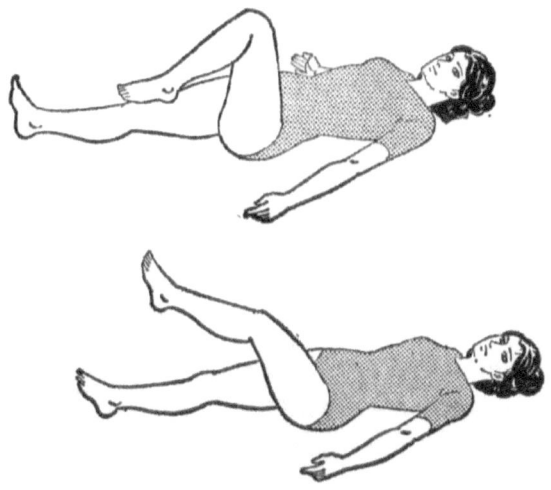

45. **Tiptoe exercises**: Wiggle your toes on both sides randomly and at the same time.

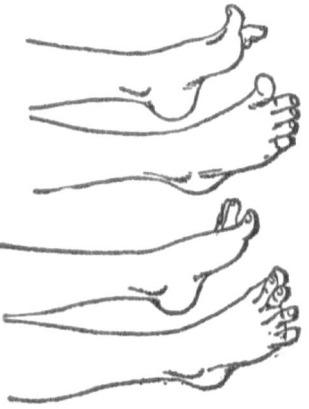

46. **Shaking the Legs**: Lie down on your back. Raise both legs together and then shake them speedily.

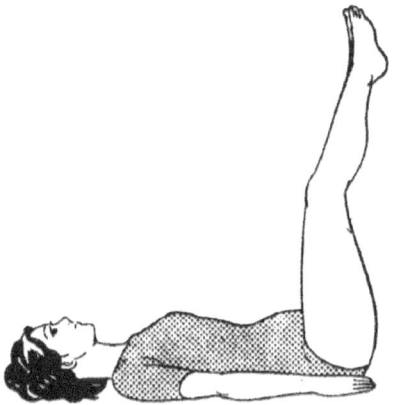

47. **Stretching the Whole Body**: Lie down on the floor, as shown in the picture, with hands up and palms outward and horizontal. Rotate ankles inward and outward and

stretch them out. At the same time, stretch the palms out.

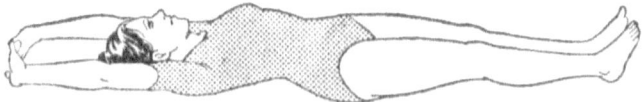

48. **Relaxation Pose**: Lie down on your back with your feet apart at shoulder width and relaxed. Put your hands out at 30 to 40 degrees from the body, palms facing up. Move slowly your head to the sides eight times. Breathe using your abdominal muscles and keep relaxed for five to ten minutes.

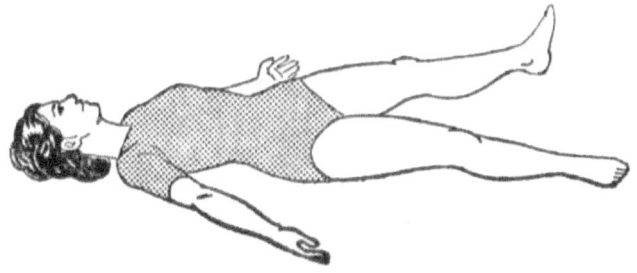

Tips for Healthy Skeletal Frame and Muscles

Squatting is healthier. Yumeiho therapy supports squatting. The therapist and the patient use mattress on the floor. No cot or bed is used to carry out Yumeiho. Therefore, Yumeiho helps not just the patient but the therapist too.

The advent of western toilets from the middle of 19th century has spread to nook and corner of the world. Earlier it was limited to royal families and disabled. The development of indoor plumbing and modernity has allowed large poorer sections of the society to use throne-like western toilets. Evacuation in the sitting posture is not complete because puborectalis muscle is strained. The puborectalis muscle, which is part of the Levator ani, relaxes allowing complete defecation only in squatting posture. Perhaps the spread of sitting on western toilets for defecation has increased the incidence of several diseases like diverticulosis, appendicitis, hemorrhoids, bladder incontinence, hiatus hernia, poorly closed ileoceacal valve leading to ileitis etc. Squatting also help empty the gall bladder and thus prevents the formation of gallstones.

Sitting on the floor improves our posture. Good posture helps prevent injuries and avoid needless pain on certain muscles. Sitting frequently on the floor also improves strength and flexibility. Moreover, this posture humbles us.

Sitting for long periods, like couch potato, can lead to several health problems. Sitting in a sofa or a comfortable chair for ten hours or more a day can wreak havoc. Sitting gives more pressure on spine than in standing. Long sitting periods can cause varicose veins, diabetes, strained neck and shoulders, risk of developing blood circulation problems for heart, impaired digestion etc. The gluteal muscle atrophy is another risk because of pressure and disuse. It may lead to low back pain, difficulty in rising from seat and climbing stairs. Sitting for long periods also leads to posterior hip tilt.

Sports and swimming definitely help you strengthen the skeletal frame and muscles of your body. On the other hand, try YumeihoBics!

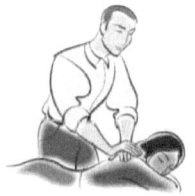

Glossary

Understanding Yumeiho therapy requires knowledge of human body and basics of medical science. Hence, some technical terms used in this book are explained here. They contain names of important diseases, terms related to human anatomy, physiology and pathology.

Angina pectoris: discomfort and chest pain due to reduction of blood supply to the cardiac muscle.
Ankylosing spondylitis: an inflammatory disease of the spine that can cause some of the vertebrae to fuse together, which makes the spine less flexible. Also known as bamboo spine.
Appendicitis: inflammation of the appendix, a vestigial organ, finger-shaped projection attached to the large intestine at the start.
Arthritis: a form of joint disorder that involves inflammation in one or more joints. There are over 100 different forms of arthritis. The most common form is osteoarthritis, a degenerative joint disease.
Atlas: the first cervical vertebra. Any dislocation or misalignment may lead to domino effect causing many unrelated problems in the musculoskeletal systaem.
Bachache: pain felt in the lower or upper back due to conditions affecting spine, ligaments, discs, spinal cord, nerves and muscles.
Biliary lithiasis: concretions formed in the gall bladder.
Bursae: A fluid-filled sac that functions as cushioning surface to reduce friction between the bones and the muscles or tendons crossing the joint.
Candidiasis: fungal infection due to any type of Cadida, known as yeast.

Cervical vertebrae: Seven bony rings that reside in neck between the base of the skull and thoracic vertebrae in thorax or trunk.

Cobb's angle: is used to quantify the magnitude of the spinal deformity in scoliosis and other injuries to spine.

Counternutation: posterior movement of the sacrum in relation to hipbones.

Diverticulosis: small pouches that bulge out from colon. This may happen in old age due to low fiber diet.

Frozen shoulder: pain and stiffness in the shoulder. It is also known as adhesive capsulitis or shoulder contracture.

Furuncle: deep folliculitis, infection of the hair follicle by the Staphylococcus aureus, also called boil.

Gout: form of acute arthritis that causes severe pain and swelling in the joints. It occurs when there are high levels of uric acid circulating in the blood, which can cause urate crystals to settle in the tissues of the joints.

Hemorrhoids: swollen veins in the anal area that may be bleeding or very painful.

Hiatus hernia: esophagus pushing down or stomach pushing up through the diaphragm muscle, that separates the thoracic cage from the abdomen.

Kyphosis: extreme curvature of the upper back, also known as a hunchback.

Laminectomy: Surgical removal of back part of the vertebrae to make room and reduce compression and pressure on the spinal cord and nerves.

Lordosis: Inward curve of the lumbar spine. An anterior concavity in the curvature of the lumbar and cervical spine as viewed from the side. A small degree of lordosis is normal.

Lumbago: lower back pain.

Lumbar vertebrae: Five spinal bones between the ribcage and pelvis.

Microdiscectomy: a minimally invasive surgical procedure in patients with herniated lumbar disc to reduce pressure on spinal nerve column.

Myocardial infarction: reduction of the blood supply to part of the cardiac muscle and its inability to respond to impulses.

Mycosis: fungal infections of skin and other parts of the body.

Neuralgia: an intense burning or stabbing pain caused by irritation of or damage to a nerve. The pain is usually brief but may be severe and feels as if it is shooting along the course of the affected nerve.

Nutation: anterior movement of the sacrum in relation to hipbones.

Osteoarthritis: a degenerative disease due to damage to cushion or cartilage in the joint leading to pain, stiffness and swelling. Also known as 'wear and tear' arthritis.

Osteitis: inflammation of the bone.

Osteoporosis: bones become very fragile and brittle; porous bone

Piriformis syndrome: compression caused by piriformis muscle, a flat, bandlike muscle located in the buttocks near the top of hip joint, on sciatic nerve. Its similar to sciatica.

Rheumatoid arthritis: an autoimmune disease that can cause chronic inflammation of the joints.

Ribs: long curved bones that create ribcage protecting lungs and heart.

Sacrum: Large triangular bone at the base of spine formed by fusion of five sacral vertebrae.

Sciatica: pain along the course of sciatic nerve extending from lower back down the back of each leg.

Scoliosis: side-to-side curvature of the spine.

Japanese Yumeiho Therapy

Sinew: see Tendon.

Spinal nerves: There are 31 pairs of spinal nerves – 8 cervical, 12 thoracic, 5 lumbar, 5 sacral and one coccygeal. They are mixed i.e. they carry sensory, motor and autonomic signal carrying fibers.

Spondylitis: inflammation of the vertebra.

Spondylolisthesis: A spinal disorder in which a vertebra (bone) slips forward onto the bone below it.

Spondylosis: Spinal degeneration accompanied by pain, usually in cervical area.

Synovial fluid: is thick viscous egg-white like fluid that fills the joints and bursae, which acts a lubricant.

Tendon: A tough band of fibrous connective tissue linking muscle to bone. They are made of collagen, a structural protein.

Thoracic vertebrae: Twelve spinal bones between cervical vertebrae and lumbar vertebrae. It is the middle segment of the spine.

Thrombophlebitis: inflammation of vein due to blood clot

Ulcertativ colitis: inflammatory bowel disease causing diarrhea and abdominal pain.

Whiplash: neck injury caused by sudden movement of the head forwards, backwards and sideways.

www.ingramcontent.com/pod-product-compliance
Lightning Source LLC
Chambersburg PA
CBHW031427210526
45464CB00005B/2081